First Aid for Horses

What to do until the veterinarian arrives

Dr. Charles H. Denning, Jr.

Illustrated by Linda L. Sale

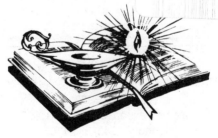

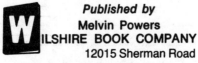

Published by
Melvin Powers
WILSHIRE BOOK COMPANY
12015 Sherman Road
No. Hollywood, California 91605
Telephone: (213) 875-1711 / (818) 983-1105

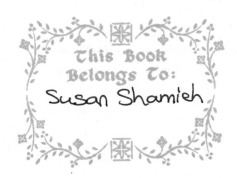

This Book
Belongs To:
Susan Shamieh

Printed by

HAL LEIGHTON PRINTING COMPANY
P.O. Box 3952
North Hollywood, California 91605
Telephone: (213) 983-1105

Library of Congress Catalog Card Number 76-181455

ISBN 0-87980-189-1

Printed in the United States of America

CONTENTS

LIST OF ILLUSTRATIONS

FIRST AID (fürst 'ād), adj. emergency treatment for injury or sudden illness given before regular medical care is available.

Dr. Charles H. Denning, Jr. has compiled this comprehensive guide to aid horseowner's throughout the world in recognizing the symptoms of various diseases and illness peculiar to horses.

The symptoms carefully described in each chapter enable the horseowners in diagnosing certain ailments so that he may obtain a veterinarian's aid before the situation becomes critical.

The remedies described for each ailment are home remedies and should not be used by the reader unless he is fully acquainted with them or has consulted a veterinarian.

This book has been published by INTERNATIONAL FARRIER'S SCHOOL, the only correspondence school for learning horseshoeing in the country. For further information, write:

INTERNATIONAL FARRIER'S SCHOOL
Box 385
Tujunga, California 91042

CHAPTER I

CONFORMATION AND POINTS – DEFECTS AND BLEMISHES

CONFORMATION AND POINTS

The forehead should be broad and not bulging; the eyes full, clear, and prominent, with a mild expression, and not showing any of the white; the muzzle not too large, as a coarse, large muzzle indicates ill breeding; the nostrils large and open; the face straight; and the lower jaw with ample width between the two sides, for the development and play of the larynx (Adam's apple) and windpipe, and, in addition, to allow the head to be nicely bent on the neck.

The ears should be of medium size, set well on the head and held erect.

The parotid and submaxillary regions should be free from large glands and without any loose skin at the lower part of the throat.

The neck should be of moderate length, clean and not too narrow at a point just in rear of the throat; a short, thick neck does not allow free movement from side to side, and a long, slim neck is apt to be too pliable. A neck with concave upper border, known as "ewe neck" is unsightly. The jugular channel or furrow should be free from enlargements. The point of the shoulder should be well developed. The point of the elbow should not be turned in, as the horse in that case is apt to turn his toes out; the opposite conformation results in the condition called "pigeontoed."

The forearm should be long and muscular; the knee broad, and when looked at from the front, much wider than the limb above and below, but tapering off backward to a comparatively thin edge. A bending of the knee backward is called a "calf knee," and is very objectionable. The opposite condition is known as "knee sprung."

The cannon should be of uniform size; if smaller just below the knee than elsewhere (a condition called "tied in"), weakness is to be expected.

The fetlock joint should be of good size and clean; the pasterns of moderate length, and forming an angle of between 45 and 50 degrees with the ground or floor.

The foot should be of moderate size; a flat foot or one too narrow at the heels is objectionable.

The relative proportions of the shoulders and the exact shape desirable vary considerably in riding and working horses. Thus, when speed and activity are essential, as in the riding horse, the shoulder should be oblique (sloping), as this shape gives elasticity to the gait of the horse. For the working horse, working in harness, a more upright shoulder bears the pressure of the collar more evenly, and when the collar is at right angle to the traces the horse exerts his strength to the greatest advantage. The front line of the shoulder must be clearly marked; an irregular surface or excessive muscular development in the region prevents a close fit of the collar.

The withers should not be thin and high, as this conformation will allow the saddle to slip too far forward and the pommel will rest upon the withers. The bars of the saddle will be forced against the shoulder blades, causing irritation and inflammation, and preventing free motion of the shoulders; the constraint causes stumbling. On the other hand, the withers should not be low or thick, as the saddle is then apt to pinch them.

1

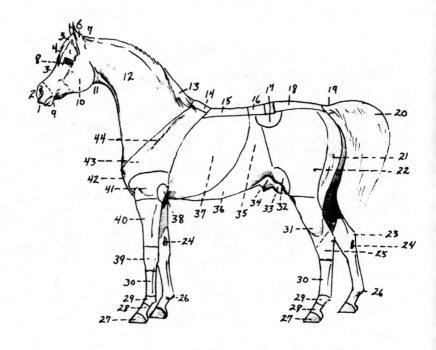

PLATE I

Points of the horse.

1.	Muzzel	16.	Loins	30.	Cannon
2.	Nostrils	17.	Point of Hip	31.	Gaskin
3.	Face	18.	Croup	32.	Stifle
4.	Forehead	19.	Dock	33.	Testicles
5.	Forelock	20.	Tail	34.	Sheath
6.	Ears	21.	Buttock	35.	Flank
7.	Poll	22.	Thigh	36.	Belly
8.	Eye	23.	Point of Hock	37.	Ribs or Barrel
9.	Chin	24.	Chestnut	38.	Elbow
10.	Jaw	25.	Hock	39.	Knee
11.	Throat	26.	Ergot	40.	Forearms
12.	Neck	27.	Hoof	41.	Arm
13.	Mane	28.	Pastern	42.	Point of Shoulder
14.	Withers	29.	Fetlock	43.	Shoulder
15.	Back			44.	Angle of Shoulder

The breast and chest should be of moderate width and have considerable depth; the narrow chest indicates weakness, and the wide, heavy chest is suitable for heavy-draft horses only.

The capacity of the lungs is marked by the size of the chest at the girth, but the stamina will depend upon the length of the back ribs. The barrel should not be broad back of the cinch, as it would cause the cinch to slip forward and chafe the body just back of the point of the elbow. The opposite conformation would allow the saddle and cinch to slip backward. The back should be short, with muscles well developed, and the upper lines of the back bending down a little behind the withers and then swelling out very gently to the junction of the loins, which can hardly be too broad and muscular.

The last rib should be placed close to the point of the hip, as this is an indication of strength, and the horse is more easily kept in good condition than one having the opposite conformation.

A slightly arched loin is essential to the power of carrying weight; the concave or "sway-back" is therefore a sign of weakness; the much arched or "roach back" is almost sure to give uneasy action from its want of elasticity.

The hips should be broad, smooth, and muscular.

The croup should be well rounded, should slope slightly downward and be of moderate length; both the straight, horizontal croup and the drooping croup are unsightly; when the croup droops and also becomes narrow below the tail, the conformation is known as "goose rump" and is a sign of weakness.

The dock should be large and muscular; the tail carried firmly and well away from the quarters.

The quarter (thigh and buttock) and gaskin should be broad. The muscles of the two quarters should come close together, leaving no hollow below the anus; the widely separate conformation is an indication of a want of constitution.

The hock should be of good size, but clean and flat, and with a good clean point standing clear of the joint. The two hocks should stand well apart, but not enough to give the horse the appearance of being "bow-legged." "Cow-hocked," so called, is when the hocks stand close together and the hind feet wide apart, with the toes turned out.

If the hocks stand in, it will be noticed that the stifles stand out, and the reverse. "Straight hock" and "crooked hock" are terms used to express the shape of the hind leg as seen from the side; both shapes are objectionable. "Sickle hock" describes the curve which results from a crooked hock, a short cannon, and a sloping pastern.

The cannon should be short, not tied in below the hock, and the line from the point of the hock to the back part of the fetlock should be straight.

The fetlock when bent forward is an indication of weakness known as "cocked ankle." The hind fetlocks, pasterns, and feet should correspond to those of the fore extremity, but the pasterns are usually more upright.

DEFECTS AND BLEMISHES

Defects and blemishes are those results of injuries (more or less severe) which show on the outside of the body. They are regarded as external diseases, and may be classed as follows:

1. Diseases of bones.
2. Diseases of synovial membranes.
3. Diseases of muscles, tendons, ligaments, and skin.
4. Diseases of the foot.

1. Diseases of bones.

Bone spavin. Location: Lower and inner part of the hock joint.
Splints. Location: Usually appearing on the inner side of the upper third of the front cannon; occasionally found on the outer side of the upper third of the hind cannon.
Sidebones. (ossification of lateral cartilages). Location: Sides of the foot just above the coronet.
Ringbone. Location: Between coronet and fetlock joint.

2. Diseases of synovial membranes.

Bog spavin. Location: Front part of hock joint.
Thorough/pin. Location: Upper and back part of hock joint.
Wind puffs (windgalls). Location: On the sides of the tendons just above the fetlock joints.

Other bursal enlargements (distended synovial sacs or pouches) may be found located on various parts of the legs, but no special name has been given to them.

3. Diseases of the muscles, tendons, ligaments, and skin.

Poll evil. Location: In the region of the poll.
Fistulous withers. Location: In the region of the withers.
Sweeny. (atrophy or wasting of the museles.) Location: Usually in the shoulder or the hip.
Broken knees. Location: Front part of the kneejoint.
Capped elbow. Location: Point of the elbow.
Capped hock. Location: Point of the hock.
Curb. Location: Lower and back part of the hock.
Sprung knees. Location: Knees.
Cocked ankles. Location: Fetlock joints.
Bowed tendons. Location: Flexor tendons below the knee and hock.
Breakdown. Location: Sprain of the suspensory ligament.
Saddle galls. Location: On the saddle bed.
Cinch galls. Location: On the parts coming in contact with the cinch.
Collar galls. Location: On the parts coming in contact with the collar.

4. Diseases of the foot.

Thrush. Location: Frog.
Canker. Location: Frog and sole.
Chronic laminitis. Location: Sensitive laminae.
Corn. Location: Between the wall and bar.
False quarter and quarter crack. Location: Quarters of the hoof.
Quittor. Location: Top of the coronet.
Contracted heels. Location: Heels.
Toe cracks. Location: At the toe of the hoof.
Seedy toe. Location: At the toe of the hoof.

CHAPTER II

STABLE MANAGEMENT OF THE SICK AND INJURED

CARE OF THE SICK

The sick horse should, if practicable, be immediately removed to a large, clean, light and well-ventilated box stall, free from drafts and located as far as possible from other horses. Clean bedding should be provided, and the stall kept free from manure and moisture. If such a stall cannot be provided, a double stall, with the kicking bar removed and ropes or bars placed across the front of it, will answer the purpose.

If the patient is suffering from a febrile disease (fever) during the cold season of the year, paulins or horse covers can be hung up in such a manner as to serve as a protection from drafts, care being taken to allow sufficient air to enter this improvised box stall. Such patients must be clothed according to the season of the year, the blanket drawn well forward on the neck and fastened in front, the legs, after hand-rubbing, bandaged with red flannels. The bandages should be changed several times daily, and the legs thoroughly rubbed to stimulate circulation.

Horses with diseases of the nervous system require to be kept absolutely quiet, and must be removed as far as possible from all noise. It is preferable that only one man be allowed to attend to their wants, as a change of attendants would very likely cause excitement and thus increase the severity of the disease. Animals suffering from debilitating diseases should be tempted with and fed any food that is rich in nourishment and easily digested. Salt should frequently be added. The food, etc., should be given only in such quantities as the animal will readily eat, and any portion left over should be at once removed, as food constantly placed before a sick animal will have a tendency to deprive it of all appetite. Food that is wet, such as bran mashes or steamed oats, will soon sour in warm weather and will get cold or may freeze during the winter; if eaten in those conditions it may cause diarrhea, colic, etc. Feed boxes, water buckets, and all parts of the stall must be kept clean and free from odor. The hay should be clean and bright, and only the best given to the sick animal. Pure water should be provided, and placed in such a position as to enable the animal to reach it without difficulty; a sick horse will frequently rinse the lips and mouth with water if given the opportunity, even when not thirsty. The water should be changed as often as necessary during the day to insure a pure and fresh supply at all times.

A horse suffering from colic requires sufficient space, well bedded, to prevent injuring himself by rolling during a spasm of pain. A man should be constantly in attendance, as there is danger that the animal may become cast and be unable to get up without assistance.

Undigested matter being the exciting cause in almost all cases of colic, food should be withheld for about twelve hours after all pain has disappeared, and then given only in small quantities during the next twenty-four hours, after which the ordinary ration may be resumed. A few swallows of pure water may be given at short intervals, but special care must be taken when the water is very cold.

The pulse is the beating of the arteries, usually felt at the jaw (the submaxillary artery), and is an important guide in determining the physical condition of the animal; the normal pulsations are about 40 per minute. The count is best taken by placing the fore or middle finger transversely on the artery. The slightest excitement, when the horse is sick, will cause an alteration in the pulse; therefore the animal should be approached very quietly. A strong and full pulse is an indication of health.

In the first stages of fever the pulse is full and bounding, afterwards becoming small and weak. A very slow pulse denotes disease or injury of the brain or spinal cord. An imperceptible pulse indicates the approach of death.

At rest the healthy horse breathes from 13 to 15 times per minute. Difficult or rapid breathing is a prominent symptom of disease of the respiratory organs; it may also be observed in some cases of flatulent colic. Abdominal breathing is the respiratory movement performed with the ribs fixed as much as possible, owing to pain or mechanical obstruction in the chest, and is a symptom of pleurisy and hydrothorax (water in the chest).

Irregular breathing is that condition where there is a want of harmonious correspondence between the inspiratory and expiratory movements, and is observed in the disease commonly known as "broken wind" or "heaves." The inspiratory movement in this affection is performed quickly and with jerky effort, while the expiratory movement is performed slowly and with a double action, more particularly of the abdominal muscles. Irregular breathing often becomes spasmodic or convulsive during the progress of the disease. The condition and color of the visible mucous membranes should be closely observed; as will be learned in detail later, they are an important guide in determining the physical condition of the animal.

The normal temperature of the horse in the internal part which is most easily accessible, the rectum, may be estimated at from 99° to 101° F. In very young animals the temperature is commonly about 101°, but in very old ones it has been known to be as low as 96° F. The temperature of the external parts of the body becomes lower according to their distance from the heart, and liable to much variation from the state of the surrounding atmosphere. Fever is an elevation of temperature.

The production of animal heat is due to certain chemical and vital changes which are continually taking place in the body; these changes consist in the absorption of oxygen by the capillaries in the lungs, and the combination of that oxygen with the carbon and hydrogen derived (first) from the disintegration of animal tissues and (second) from certain elements of the food which have not been converted into tissue.

This combination with oxygen, or oxidation, not only takes place in the blood, which may be looked upon as a fluid tissue, but in the tissue cells also, in all parts of the body, the animal heat being maintained by the natural changes which are essential to a healthy condition.

As previously stated, oxygen is absorbed from the air by the capillaries of the lungs in respiration (breathing). Expired air is found to have lost about 10 per cent of the oxygen contained in pure air, and to have accumulated a like amount of a combination of carbon and oxygen, called carbonic acid gas. If we imagine the animal breathing and rebreathing the same air, it can be seen that the oxygen, so necessary for the purification of the blood, would soon diminish to a dangerous degree. Hence, we realize the importance of a large supply of air to draw on and the necessity of good ventilation. At each inspiration the horse draws about 250 cubic inches of air into the lungs, and he therefore requires about 2 cubic feet per minute, or 120 per hour. It is customary, in building ordinary stables, to allow 1,600 cubic feet of air space (over twelve hours' supply) for each animal, and to provide means of admitting fresh air without causing drafts. In recooperation stables the allowance is increased to 1,900 cubic feet.

6

Without good air the blood is imperfectly purified, the vitality of the animal is lessened, he is more susceptible to disease, and will succumb more easily when attacked; consequently horses should never be kept in the vicinity of a marsh, the air from which contains an excess of carbonic acid gas and a diminished supply of the necessary oxygen.

CARE OF THE INJURED

If the horse is seriously injured and stands with difficulty, he should be placed in slings to partially support the weight of the body. The slings must be properly adjusted, fitting closely behind the elbows in such a manner as to support the weight of the body on the chest and not on the abdomen. This position is maintained by the use of the breast piece and breeching, which prevent the shifting of the sling. A single stall, having a level floor, free from bedding, is more suitable than one allowing more motion to the animal.

If the horse is but slightly injured, there is no necessity of placing him in slings. An ordinary stall with a level floor is all that is required. After the injury has been dressed he should be allowed to stand without being disturbed. If very lame, and movement is painful, the more quiet he is kept the more quickly will recovery take place. Absolute rest and perfect quietude are two very essential things, and when secured they will hasten the process of recovery without inflicting unnecessary pain upon the animal. In some surgical cases it is necessary to restrain the animal so that he cannot injure himself by rubbing or biting the affected parts. This can be accomplished by tying up the head or by the application of side lines. Bandages may be applied to the legs of animals for different purposes: First, to give support to the blood vessels and synovial bursae; second, to dry and warm the legs; third, to support packs used in applying hot and cold lotions; and fourth, when conditions are favorable, to check hemorrhages.

WATER SUPPLY

However harmless impure water may have been to animals in a wild state, the more we subject them to an artificial existence the more we remove them from the immunity they may have possessed against common causes of disease and the greater liability is there for the development of diseases which originally may never have existed. In other words, the domesticated animal should always have pure water; when the vitality is further reduced by sickness the necessity of absolute purity is even more imperative.

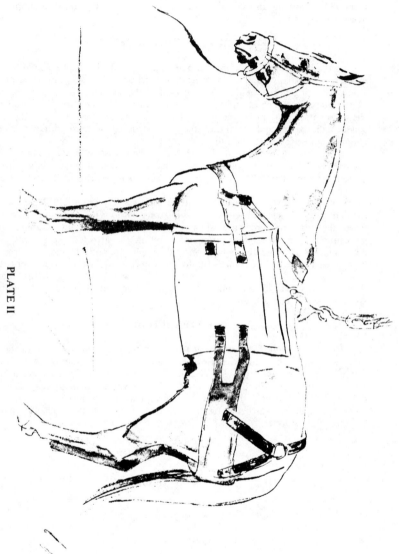

PLATE II

The horse in slings.

CHAPTER III

ANATOMY

Anatomy is a description of the structures that make up the body.

The Skeleton

The skeleton is the framework for the support of the softer structures, and is composed of 216 bones (exclusive of the teeth) of various sizes and forms.

Flat bones, such as the skull, ribs, and scapula, are found covering vital organs; long bones are found principally in the extremities, for the support of the body.

The spinal column is composed of bones of very irregular shape, which are divided into five groups according to their location, and are known as *vertebrae*. Commencing at the back of the head, the first seven are called the *cervical* vertebrae, or bones of the neck; of these the first is called *atlas*, the second *axis*; the next eighteen are called the *dorsal* vertebrae, forming the main part of the back; the next six, the *lumbar* vertebrae, form the loins; the croup or *sacrum* is composed of five bones, which in the adult animal are united together as one bone; and following this are found the *coccygeal* or tail bones, numbering from thirteen to twenty. All vertebrae have irregular projections of varying length, called *spinous processes*; these are named, according to location, dorsal, cervical, etc.; the third to sixth dorsal spinous processes (often called dorsal spines) are very long and form the withers.

The ribs are eighteen on each side, attached above to the dorsal vertebrae. The first eight (true or fixed ribs) are attached below, by cartilage, to the *sternum* or breastbone; the remaining ten (false or floating ribs) are attached by cartilage to one another and indirectly to the sternum; they form the walls of the chest and serve as a protection for the heart, lungs, and large blood vessels.

The skull, containing cavities (or chambers), is composed of irregularly shaped flat bones, the most important of which is the *cranium*, or brainpan, occupied by the brain and communicating with the bony canal (containing the *spinal cord*), which passes through the center of the cervical, dorsal, lumbar, sacral, and sometimes the first two or three coccygeal vertebrae. The *orbital cavities* (containing the eyes) communicate with the brain by narrow passages, through one of which the *optic nerve* passes.

On each side, below the eye, are two closed cavities known as the *superior* (upper) and *inferior* (lower) *maxillary sinuses*; in the lower third of the skull are found the nasal chambers extending from the nostrils backward to the *pharynx*, and separated by a thin partition of bone and cartilage, called the *septum nasi*; the floor of these chambers forms the roof of the mouth. From the orbital cavities the skull gradually becomes narrower and terminates a short distance below the nostrils in the *premaxilla*, which contains the six upper *incisor* teeth; these six, with the corresponding teeth in the lower jaw, form the *anterior* (front) boundary of the mouth, which extends back to the pharynx. On the upper portion of the back of the mouth cavity are found six *molar* or grinder teeth on each side; that portion of the jaw between them and the incisors is called the *interdental space*. Situated on each side near the incisor teeth in this space are found, in the male, and rarely in the female, the *tushes* or canine teeth.

The *inferior maxilla* or lower jaw is composed of two segments firmly united in front and spreading backward somewhat in the form of a letter V. Each branch, at

9

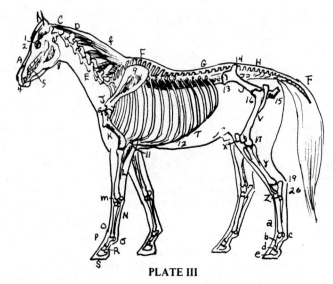

PLATE III

Skeleton of the horse.

A. Head
B. Lower Jaw
C. Atlas
D. Axis
E. The remaining five cervical vertebrae
F. Spinous processes of the back and withers
G. Lumbar vertebrae
H. Sacrum
I. Coccygeal, or tail bones
J. Scapula, or shoulder blade
K. Humerus, or arm bone
L. Radius and ulna or bones of the forearm
M. Carpal, or Knee Bones
N. Small metacarpal, or splint bone
O. Large Metascarpal, or cannon bone
P. Os suffraginis, or pastern bone
Q. Sesamoid bones
R. Os coronae, or lower pastern bone
S. Os pedis, or coffin bone
T. Ribs
U. Pelvis
V. Femur, or thigh bone
X. Patella, or stifle bone
Y. Tibia and fibula, or leg bones
Z. Tarsal, or hock bone

a. Large metatarsal, or cannon bone
b. Upper pastern bone
c. Sesamoid bones
d. Lower pastern bone
e. Coffin bone
f. Ligamentum nuchae, or neck ligament

1. Cranium
2. Orbital cavity
4. Incisor teeth
5. Molar teeth
6. Shoulder joint
9. Cartilage of porlongation
11. Ulna, or elbow bone
12. Rib cartilages
13. Point of the hip; outer angle of the ilium
14. Point of the croup; inner angle of the ilium
15. Ischium
16. Hip joint
17. Stifle joint
19. Calcaneum
20. Cuboid

10

the end, turns upward and is united to the skull proper in a movable joint. The branches of the jaw include a space appropriately called the maxillary space. Located in the united or front part of this bone are the inferior incisors and canine teeth, and, in the branches, the inferior molars, which correspond to those of the upper jaw. The space between the molars and incisors is the same as that in the upper jaw.

The front leg is composed of the following bones, named in order from above downward: *Scapula*, shoulder blade; *humerus*, bone of the arm; *radius*, bone of the forearm; and *ulna*, bone of the elbow (radius and ulna are united in one bone); *carpus*, knee bones (seven small bones); *large metacarpal*, cannon bone; two *small metacarpals*, splint bones (the three metacarpal bones are joined together, forming the *metacarpus*); two *sesamoids*, pulley bones; *os suffraginis*, upper pastern bone; *os coronae*, lower pastern bone; *os pedis*, coffin bone; and *os navicularis*, shuttle bone. The scapula is extended by means of a thin plate of gristle, called the *"cartilage of prolongation,"* which offers additional attachment for the muscles of the body.

The *pelvis* is composed of two segments. In each segment are three united, irregularly shaped, flat bones, namely, *ilium, ischium,* and *pubis* (haunch bones). The ischium and pubis bones are also united in pairs, forming the floor of the pelvic cavity occupied by the bladder and rectum. The two ilium bones or branches are triangular in shape. The outer angle in each case is the *point of the hip*. The two inner angles are close to each other, and together form the *point of the croup*. Just below this point each branch is attached to the sacrum by ligaments. That portion of the ilium extending back to the hip joint is called the "shaft."

The hind leg is composed of the following bones: *Femur*, thigh bone; *tibia*, leg bone; *fibula*, accessory leg bone; *patella*, stifle bone; *tarsus*, hock (made up of six small bones, named *calcaneum, astragalus, cuneiform magnum, medium* and *parvum*, and *cuboid*); *large metatarsal*, cannon bone; two *small metatarsals*, splint bones. Below the cannon, the bones have the same name as in the fore leg.

JOINTS

A joint is a movable union between two or more bones. Covering the adjacent surfaces in the joint is a thin and very smooth layer of a peculiar kind of cartilage called *articular cartilage*. A lubricating fluid, *synovia*, joint oil, is required to reduce the amount of friction; this fluid is secreted or formed by the synovial membrane and the latter is confined and protected by the *capsular ligament* which completely surrounds the joint. Outside of the capsular ligament are binding ligaments holding the bones in position.

The joints of the foreleg are as follows: *Shoulder joint*, formed by the lower end of the scapula and the head of the humerus; *elbow joint*, by the radius, ulna, and humerus; *knee joint*, by the radius, seven small bones (carpals), and the upper end of the metacarpals; *fetlock joint*, by the large cannon, upper pastern bone, and the two sesamoids; *pastern joint*, by the upper and lower pastern bones; *coffin joint*, by the lower pastern, coffin bone, and shuttle bone.

The following joints make up the articulation of the hind leg: *Hip joint*, formed by the socket of the pelvis and the head of the femur; *stifle joint*, by the lower end of the femur, head of the tibia, and the patella; *hock joint*, by the lower end of the tibia, six small bones (tarsals), and the upper ends of the metatarsals. The fetlock, pastern, and coffin joints correspond to those of the fore limb.

11

LIGAMENTS

Ligaments are, generally speaking, strong bands of white fibrous inelastic tissue. Their principal use is to firmly bind joints together, thereby preventing vibration and diminishing friction.

The suspensory ligament should be carefully studied on account of the numerous accidents to which it is liable. It is a long, strong band of fibrous tissue originating in the back part of the lower bones of the knee and in the upper part of the cannon bone; it occupies the space between the splint bones and passes down immediately behind the cannon bone, lying between it and the tendon (sinew) of the *flexor pedis perforans*: it bifurcates (divides into two) opposite the lower third of the cannon bone and becomes attached to the sesamoids, whence the parts pass forward and downward, joining the tendon of the *extensor pedis* just above the pastern joint. It is thin and comparatively weak near the knee, but as it approaches the fetlock joint it almost equals the back tendons in substance, and its size and wiriness to the touch may be taken as some test of the power of any particular leg to resist a breakdown.

The suspensory ligament of the hind leg corresponds in every particular to that of the fore leg.

The calcaneo-cuboid ligament stretches from the posterior (back) border of the calcaneum to the posterior part of the cuboid, ending on the head of the external (outer) splint bone. A sprain of this ligament is known as a *"curb."*

Capsular ligaments, as we have seen, are pouch-shaped, are found around joints, and are intended to protect the lubricating apparatus inside.

Some ligaments are made up almost entirely of yellow tissue, which is elastic. The *ligamentum nuchae*, neck ligament, is an important example. It occupies the space in front of the dorsal spines, above the cervical vertebrae, and is attached to the top of the skull. In this position it separates the neck muscles of the right side from those of the left. The object of elasticity in this ligament is to permit great freedom in the motion of the head, although supporting its great weight in proper position.

MUSCLES AND TENDONS

The muscles are divided into voluntary and involuntary muscles; the former being under the direct control of the will, as, for example, the muscles of the neck, legs, tail, etc.; and the latter acting independently of the animal's will, as, for example, the heart, intestinal muscles, etc.

The muscles form about one-half of the entire weight of the body. With regard to their form they are divided into long, wide, and short. Long muscles are generally found in the limbs; wide muscles are stretched beneath the skin or around the great cavities of the trunk, and short muscles are found chiefly around the irregularly shaped bones.

Tendons are white, round or flattened cords affixed to the extremities of long muscles, attaching them to other structures, but themselves neither stretching nor contracting.

All leg muscles are long muscles. *Extensors* are those that have the power of straightening the limb; *flexors*, of bending the limb.

The *extensor pedis* is the principal extensor of the fore leg; it originates at the lower extremity of the humerus, and its fleshy portion continues to the lower third of the *radius*; at this point it becomes tendinous, and, passing down over the knee,

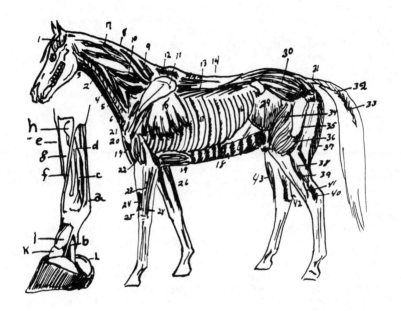

PLATE IV

Muscles and tendons of the horse.

a. Flexor pedis perforatus tendon
b. Flexor pedis perforans tendon
c. Suspensory ligament
d. Check ligament
e. Extensor pedis tendon
f. Extensor suffraginis tendon
g. Cannon bone
h. Splint bone
i. Upper pastern bone
k. Lower pastern bone
l. Lateral cartilage

14. Logissimus dorsi
21. Flexor brachii
23. Extensor suffraginis
24. Extensor metacarpi magnus
25. Extensor pedis tendon
26. Flexor pedis perforans
30. Gluteus maximus
38. Gastrocnemius externus
39. Flexor pedis perforatus
40. Flexor pedis perforans
41. Peroneus
42. Flexor metatarsi
43. Extensor pedis

continues along the front of the leg and becomes attached to the upper and front part of the os pedis. Action, to extend the foot.

The *extensor suffraginis* has its origin from the external head and outer border of the radius and from the side of the ulna; it is inserted (attached) to the upper front part of the os suffraginis. Action, to extend the foot.

The *extensor metacarpi magnus* has its origin from the lower and external surface of the humerus, passes down the front of the radius and kneejoint, and is attached to the upper end of the large metacarpal bone. Action, to extend the metacarpus.

The *flexor brachii* has its origin from the lower end of the scapula, near the shoulder joint, and passes down in front of that joint and the humerus and becomes attached to the upper front part of the radius. Action, to flex the elbow joint and extend the shoulder.

The *flexor pedis perforatus* originates from the inner and lower part of the humerus; it passes down the back of the leg, becoming tendinous just above the carpus; behind the pastern it bifurcates, forming a ring for the passage of the tendon of the perforans and becomes attached to the sides of the os coronae. Action, to bend or flex the knee, fetlock, and pastern.

The *flexor pedis perforans* originates with the perforatus; its fleshy portion passes down and is attached to the back part of the radius; its tendinous portion, beginning at the knee, passes down the leg between the cannon gone and the tendon of the perforatus, over the back of the fetlock, through the arch formed by the division of the tendon of the perforatus, and is attached to the under surface of the os pedis. Action, to flex the knee and all joints below.

The *extensor pedis* of the hind leg originates from the lower and front part of the femur; its fleshy portion extends downward along the front surface of the tibia to the hock, where it becomes tendinous; passing thence down the front of the leg it is attached in the same manner as the extensor pedis of the front leg. Action, to extend the leg and flex the hock.

The *peroneus* has its origin from the external ligament of the stifle and from the outer part of the fibula, and is attached to the tendon of the extensor pedis a short distance below the hock. Action, to assist the extensor pedis.

The tendon of the peroneus is cut in the operation for *string halt*.

The *flexor metatarsi* is divided into two portions – a muscular and a tendinous. The tendinous part is a strong pearl-white cord, situated between the muscular portion and the extensor pedis. It commences at the lower extremity of the femur, and terminates in two branches – a large one inserted in front of the upper extremity of the cannon bone and a small one deviating outward to reach the front surface of the cuboid bone. The fleshy portion originates on the front face of the tibia and is inserted by two tendons, one in the head of the large metatarsal bone, the other in the small cuneiform on the inner side of the hock. Action, to flex the hock.

The *flexor pedis perforatus* of the hind leg originates at the back and lower part of the femur. Its fleshy portion extends about halfway down the tibia, then becomes tendinous, and passes over the point of the hock, continues down the back of the leg, and is attached in the same manner as the perforatus of the front leg. Action, to extend the hock and to flex the fetlock and pastern.

The *gastrocnemius externus* has a double origin at the lower and back part of the femur and is attached to the point of the hock. At the back part of the leg the tendon of this muscle becomes closely associated with the tendon of the flexor pedis perforatus, the two forming the *tendon of Achilles*, or *hamstring*.

14

The *flexor pedis perforans* of the hind leg originates at the upper and back portion of the tibia. Above the hock it becomes tendinous and passing down over the inner and back side of the hock is attached to the os pedis in the same manner as the perforans of the front limb. Action, to extend the hock and to flex the joints below.

Wide muscles are attached to other structures by broad bands of strong white tissue instead of by tendons.

The *panniculus carnosus* (fly shaker) is a wide flat muscle situated on the inner surface of the skin and covering most of the neck, sides of the chest, and belly. Action, to shake the skin.

The principal muscles of the back, loins, and haunches are the *longissimus dorsi, gluteus externus, gluteus maximus*, and *gluteus internus*.

The *longissimus dorsi* is situated on the upper part of the back and loins, and is the largest and most powerful muscle in the body, occupying the space on either side of the dorsal and lumbar spines. It is broad and fleshy at its origin in the loins and becomes narrower as it proceeds forward. It is attached to the front part of the pelvis (ilium), first two bones of the sacrum, all of the lumbar and dorsal vertebrae, the external surface of the last fifteen or sixteen ribs, and to the last three or four cervical vertebrae. Action: It is brought powerfully into play in kicking or rearing; it elevates the hind or fore quarters, according as the fore or hind limbs are on the ground. Acting on one side only, it bends the back and loins laterally.

Gluteus externus is a V-shaped muscle situated on the upper and outer part of the haunch. It originates on the front part of the ilium and at the second and third sacral spines. Insertion, to the upper and outer part of the femur. Action, to draw the thigh outward.

Gluteus maximus is a very large muscle, originating in the lumbar region; it is attached to the ilium and sacrum and is inserted on the upper and outer portion of the femur. Action, to extend the femur on the pelvis, and when the posterior limbs are fixed, to assist in rearing.

Gluteus internus is situated underneath the gluteus maximus and above the hip joint. It originates from the shaft (lower angle) of the ilium and is inserted by a tendon to the upper part of the femur. Action, to draw the leg outward and rotate it inward.

THE RESPIRATORY SYSTEM

The organs of respiration are the nostrils, nasal chambers, *pharynx, larynx, trachea, bronchi,* bronchial tubes, and air cells. All of these organs, except the air cells, are lined with a soft tissue called *mucous membrane*; where organs open to the external surface the mucous membrane and the skin are continuous. The nostrils are two oblong openings (right and left) situated in the front part of the muzzle. The nasal chambers extend from the nostrils to the pharynx and are separated from each other by the cartilaginous septum nasi; each chamber is divided by the *turbinated bone* into three passages, all lined with a delicate rose-colored mucous membrane, called the *Schneiderian membrane*, which is continuous with the skin of the nostrils.

The *pharynx* is a muscular, membranous cavity, common to the digestive and respiratory canals, somewhat cylindrical in form, and extending back to the larynx and the *esophagus*.

The *larynx* (commonly known as "Adam's apple") is a complex musculo-cartilaginous box, situated in the back part of the maxillary space, and at the front part of the trachea or windpipe. It gives passage to air and at the same time is the

15

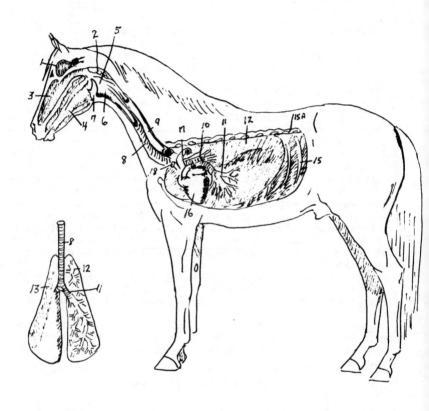

PLATE V

Respiratory apparatus.

3. Nasal chamber
4. Tongue
5. Pharynx
6. Larynx
7. Epiglottis, or potlid
8. Trachea, or windpipe
9. Esophagus or gullet
10. Section of left bronchus
11. Ramifications of the right bronchus

12. Right lung
13. Left lung, seen from above
14. Sternum
15. Ribs
15a. Section of the left ribs
16. Heart
17. Posterior aorta (Cut off)
18. Anterior aorta (Cut off)

organ of voice. The front extremity opens into the pharynx and the posterior into the trachea; the front opening is guarded by a valve called the *epiglottis* or "pot-lid," which closes mechanically in the act of swallowing and thus prevents the passage of food or water into the trachea and lungs.

The *trachea*, or windpipe, is a cylindrical, flexible tube consisting of a series of incomplete cartilaginous rings, numbering from forty to fifty, according to the length of the neck. It succeeds the larynx, runs down the neck, enters the *thorax* or chest, and terminates at the base of the heart where it branches into the right and left *bronchi*, which enter the lungs and subdivide into branches termed bronchial tubes. These, becoming gradually smaller as they divide, finally terminate in air cells. The entire ramification, when isolated, has the appearance of a tree, the trachea being the trunk, the bronchi and bronchial tubes the branches, and the air cells the leaves. These structures are accompanied throughout by arteries, veins, and nerves.

The *thorax*, or chest, is formed by the ribs, sternum, the bodies of the dorsal vertebrae, the muscles between the ribs (intercostal), and the diaphragm. It contains the lungs, heart, large blood vessels, the trachea, esophagus, and a number of nerves. The thorax is lined by two *serous membranes*, the right and left *pleura*, each pleura lining one-half the thorax and enveloping the structure contained therein. A serous membrane is a thin glistening structure and lines a closed cavity.

The lungs, the essential organs of respiration, are light, spongy organs of a conical shape, situated in the thoracic cavity. (Healthy lungs float in water.)

The *diaphragm* or midriff is the muscular partition which separates the thorax from the *abdominal cavity* or belly.

DIGESTIVE ORGANS

The digestive organs consist of the *mouth, pharynx, esophagus, stomach, intestines,* and *anus,* all lined with mucous membrane. Together they form the alimentary canal through which the alimentary matter (food) is subjected to the special actions which adapt it to the purpose of nutrition.

The mouth is an irregular cavity, containing the organs of taste and the instruments of *mastication* (chewing or grinding). It is situated between the jaws, its long diameter following that of the head, and is pierced by two openings   the anterior, for the introduction of food, and the posterior, through which the food passes into the pharynx. It is bounded in front by the lips and laterally by the cheeks; the roof is formed by the *hard palate*; the floor is occupied by the tongue, while the rear boundary is the *soft palate*. Opening into the mouth are ducts leading from the *salivary* glands: the *parotid, submaxillary,* and *sublingual* glands. The mucous membrane covers the whole free surface of the mouth and its accessories except the teeth. The lips are the organs of touch as well as of *prehension* (picking up). The soft palate is a curtain suspended between the mouth and the pharynx, attached above to the *palatine arch* (the back part of the hard palate); the lower border is free and rests on the floor of the pharynx. Owing to the great size of this curtain, the horse is unable to breathe through his mouth.

The tongue is a movable muscular organ, situated on the floor of the mouth between the branches of the lower jaw. It is the special organ of taste and at the same time assists in mastication.

The *pharynx* has been previously described.

The *esophagus*, or gullet, is a muscular tube connecting the pharynx to the stomach.

17

The *stomach* is a pear-shaped organ situated in the abdominal cavity, close to the diaphragm. Its internal, or mucous, coat is divided into right and left portions, the left is the *cuticular* portion and is continuous with the mucous membrane of the esophagus, which it resembles in structure and appearance, being of a pale white color. The right portion, the *villous*, or true digestive coat, is reddish in color, soft, very vascular (filled with blood vessels) and velvety looking; it contains the *peptic glands* which secrete *gastric juice*.

The capacity of the stomach of the horse (from 3 to 3½ gallons) is small in proportion to his size.

The intestines are divided into large and small. The small intestines are continuous with the stomach, rather more than an inch in diameter and about 72 feet in length. The large intestines, measuring about 22 feet in length, extend from the termination of the small intestines to the anus, and may be regarded as consisting of four parts, the *caecum, great colon, floating colon,* and the *rectum.*

The membranous lining of the intestines is covered with small projections called *villi*, which absorb the nourishing parts of the food. The villi are more numerous in the small intestines than in the large.

The intestines are supported throughout their entire length by strong bands of fibrous tissue (the mesentery) extending from the backbone. The mesentery is a part of the peritoneum.

The *anus* is the posterior opening of the alimentary canal and lies below the root of the tail. It forms a round projection, which becomes less prominent with age.

The *liver* is the largest secreting organ in the body, weighing from 10 to 12 pounds. It is situated immediately behind the diaphragm and in front of the stomach. The liver secretes a fluid, called bile or gall, which is emptied directly into the small intestines, as the horse is not provided with a gall bladder.

The *pancreas* (sweetbread) is situated behind the stomach and in front of the kidneys. It is of reddish cream color, and weighs about 17 ounces. Its function is to secrete pancreatic fluid, which is poured into the small intestine.

The *spleen* is situated on the left side of the stomach. It is pointed at the lower end and gradually widens as it extends up to the region of the left kidney. The spleen is of a reddish-gray color and in the healthy horse weighs from 2 to 4 pounds. In disease, however, it may reach an enormous size.

The function of the spleen is not positively known, but it is believed that this organ acts as a storehouse for the supply of blood to the stomach during digestion and that it effects some change in the blood, many authorities claiming that it forms the white blood corpuscles. (See "Blood.")

The abdominal cavity is a large, somewhat oval cavity, bounded above by the muscles of the back, below by the abdominal muscles, and in front by the diaphragm; behind it is continuous with the pelvic cavity. The cavity is lined throughout by a serous membrane called the *peritoneum.*

PHYSIOLOGY OF DIGESTION

By physiology is meant a description of the functions or uses of certain structures. The physiology of digestion describes the functions of parts of the digestive apparatus.

Food, as it passes through the digestive or alimentary canal, is subjected to a series of mechanical and chemical agencies by which it is, in greater or less part, digested and worked up to a condition in which it can be absorbed by the appropriate vessels, and, while this portion is taken up by the circulation, the effete (worthless) remainder passes on and is discharged.

The food is taken into the mouth by the lips *(prehension)*, where it is ground up *(mastication)*, and is mixed with *saliva*. Saliva, secreted by the salivary glands in different parts of the head, acts chemically upon the starchy components (parts) of the food and converts them into sugar, which is more readily absorbed. This step is called *insalivation*.

The next step, *deglutition* or swallowing, is mechanically performed by the tongue, pharynx, and esophagus.

When the food reaches the stomach it is subjected to the next step, *maceration*, a mechanical rolling, mixing, and soaking with the gastric juice. During maceration the gastric juice acts chemically upon other components (*nitrogenous* parts), rendering them absorbable. Food in the condition in which it leaves the stomach is called *chyme*.

In the small intestines the villi take up the absorbable parts already prepared, and the remaining nourishing parts are immediately subjected to the chemical action of the bile and pancreatic fluid. Chyme, acted upon by these juices, becomes *chyle*. Passing through the great length of the small intestines, nearly all of the nourishing parts of the chyle are absorbed, and the residue (remainder) enters the caecum, which is the water reservoir. (Water remains in the stomach of the horse only a short time and then passes promptly through the small intestines into the caecum.)

The residue, soaked in water, gives up, in its passage through to the rectum, the small amount of nutritive matter that has not previously been absorbed. By means of muscular cross ridges in the floating colon the effete material is mechanically molded into pellets of dung, which are stored in the rectum, whence they are ejected, at intervals, through the anus. The ejection is called *defecation*.

URINARY SYSTEM

The organs of this system secrete effete material in the form of a watery fluid, called *urine*, and expel it from the body *(urination)*. They are the *kidneys, ureters, bladder*, and *urethra*, all lined with mucous membrane.

The *kidneys* are two in number, right and left, situated on either side of the spine, immediately below the lumbar vertebrae. Their action is to secrete the urine from the blood by a process of filtering. Each kidney has a tube or duct, called the *ureter*, which carries the urine to the storage reservoir, the *bladder*. This muscular organ, by contraction, discharges the urine, at intervals, through a tube called the *urethra*, which extends to the head of the *penis*.

The normal amount of urine secreted in twenty-four hours and expelled through the penis varies from 3 to 6 quarts. The color in health is yellowish.

CIRCULATION

The organs which convey the blood throughout the body are the *heart, arteries, capillaries,* and *veins*.

The *heart* is a hollow organ, made up of involuntary muscles, and inclosed in a serous sac called *pericardium*; it is situated between the lungs, in the thoracic cavity, and averages about 6½ pounds in weight. It is divided into two parts, right and left, separated by a muscular wall. Each part contains two cavities, one above the other,

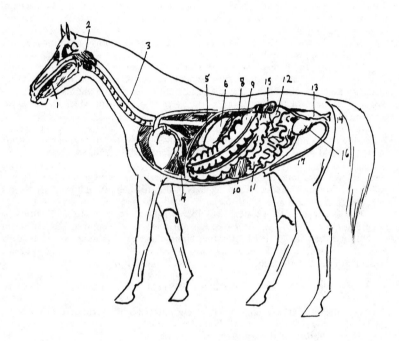

PLATE VI
Digestive apparatus.

1. Mouth
2. Pharynx
3. Esophagus
4. Diaphragm
5. Spleen
6. Stomach (left sac).
8. Liver, upper extremity
9. Large colon

10. Caecum
11. Small intestine
12. Floating colon
13. Rectum
14. Anus
15. Left kidney and its ureter
16. Bladder
17. Urethra

the upper called the *auricle* and the lower the *ventricle*. The cavities are connected by openings, which are guarded by valves to prevent a back flow of the blood.

Arteries are hollow structures or tubes, conveying the blood away from the heart, and *veins* are similar structures, bringing it back to the heart. The walls of the tubes are thicker in arteries than in veins. Veins have valves; arteries have none. Veins as well as arteries branch off and diminish in size as they extend from the heart.

The smallest arteries are connected with the smallest veins by minute vessels called *capillaries*, which are to be found in the tissue throughout the body. They are too small to be seen with the naked eye.

Blood.

The blood is a fluid which is the medium by which nutritive material is conveyed to all tissues of the body. It is an opaque, thickish, clammy fluid, with a peculiar odor and sickly, saline (salty) taste. Its color varies in different parts of the same animal, that in the arteries being a bright red or scarlet, while that in the veins is a dark purple.

Blood is composed of red blood corpuscles, or cells, and white blood corpuscles, floating in a watery liquid called *serum*, which contains the nutrient material absorbed by digestion, and certain salts.

The red cells convey the oxygen, and their presence in countless numbers gives the bright-red color to the fluid. The white corpuscles act as a protection to all parts of the body in case of disease or injury; they assist in the repair of injured tissue and destroy or check invading germs. Blood cells can be seen only with the aid of the microscope.

Circuit of the blood.

The heart, from the action of its involuntary muscles, may be likened to a force pump. The blood from the veins, *venous* or impure blood, entering the right auricle of the heart, is pumped into the right ventricle and thence through the *pulmonary artery* (lung artery) into the lungs.

In the lungs the pulmonary artery branches into small arteries and then into capillaries which surround the air cells. Here the blood gives off carbonic acid gas and receives its purifying supply of oxygen. The purified blood passes from the capillaries into the small veins, which unite in the *pulmonary veins* leading back to the left auricle.

The *arterial*, pure, or bright-red blood is then pumped into the left ventricle and thence into the arteries, small arteries, and capillaries. In these last vessels it gives up the oxygen supply to the tissues and receives the impure carbonic acid gas, which causes it to change color. The dark impure blood is then collected through the small veins into the larger veins and thence into the right auricle from which it started. This round or circuit, which is constantly going on, gives rise to the name circulation.

It has been stated that arteries convey the blood away from the heart and that veins return it. In supplying the body, arteries carry pure blood and veins carry impure blood. When, however, the impure blood is sent to the lungs for purification, it is conveyed in an artery and the pure blood returns in a vein. These *two important exceptions* must be carefully noted.

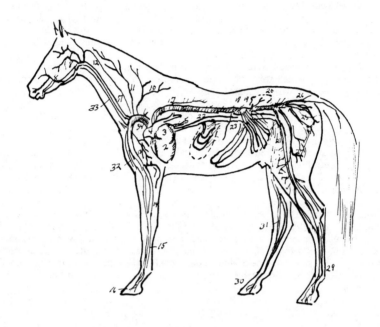

PLATE VII

Circulatory apparatus.

Note. – The left fore leg has been removed to show the vessels on
the inner side of the right leg.

1.	Heart (right ventricle)	18.	Branches distributed to the stomach,
2.	Heart (left ventricle)		spleen, pancreas, etc.
3.	Heart (left auricle)	19.	Branches distributed to the intestine
3a.	Heart (right auricle)	20.	Branch to the kidneys
4.	Pulmonary arteries (cut off)	22.	Posterior vena cava
5.	Pulmonary veins (cut off)	24.	External iliac artery
6.	Anterior aorta	25.	Internal iliac artery
7.	Common carotid artery	27.	Femoral artery
9.	Left brachial artery	28.	Posterior tibial artery
13.	Humeral artery	29.	Metatarsal artery
14.	Radial artery	30.	Venous network of the foot
15.	Metacarpal artery	33.	Jugular vein
16.	Digital artery	34.	Anterior vena cava
17.	Posterior aorta		

Arterial ramification.

The large artery given off from the left ventricle of the heart is the *common aorta*, which passes upward and forward for 2 or 3 inches and divides into the *anterior aorta* and the *posterior aorta*, supplying, respectively, the fore and hind portions of the body.

The *anterior aorta* is very short (1 or 2 inches), passes upward and forward under the trachea and between the lungs, and divides into the right and left *brachial arteries*, each supplying blood to one of the fore limbs and its neighboring muscles.

The *right brachial* artery gives off a large branch, called the common carotid. There is no corresponding branch of the left brachial. The common carotid is short and immediately divides into two branches, *right* and *left carotids*, which pass up the neck, at first under the trachea and then on either side; they follow the trachea to the throat, where they divide into branches, supplying the head.

The *brachial arteries* continue toward the front part of the thorax, winding around the first ribs, and divide into branches, supplying the fore limbs. The main branch of each is here named the *humeral artery*.

The *humeral artery* descends along the inner side of the humerus, and just above the elbow joint divides into the *anterior* and *posterior radial arteries*.

The *anterior radial* descends over the front surface of the elbow joint, passes down in front of the radius, and approaches the knee below the extensor pedis muscle, where it divides into numerous branches, supplying blood to the surrounding tissues. The *posterior radial* is a continuation of the humeral artery, passing down the inner side of the fore leg, inclining back and dividing at the lower end of the radius into the *large* and *small metacarpal arteries*.

The *small metacarpal* passes outward from the inner and back part of the knee, and, running downward, supplies nourishment to the surrounding tissues. The *large metacarpal* is a continuation of the posterior radial. It runs down the back of the knee, in company with the flexor tendon; above the fetlock it passes between the tendon and the suspensory ligament, dividing into the *external* and *internal digital arteries*, which supply the foot.

The study of the digital arteries will be taken up later, when the student has a more extended knowledge of the bones and of the elastic and sensitive structures of the foot.

We will now return to the posterior aorta. The *posterior aorta* is larger and longer than the anterior. It begins at about the level of the fourth dorsal vertebra, passes upward and backward, and reaches the left side of the spine just below the sixth or seventh dorsal vertebra. It then passes straight back into the abdominal cavity and terminates in the lumbar region below the last lumbar vertebra. During its passage to this point it gives off branches to the muscles of the ribs, to the lungs for their nourishment, to the abdominal organs, and to the muscles of the loins. Below the last lumbar vertebra it divides into four branches, the *right* and *left external* and *internal iliacs*, which supply blood to the hind extremities.

The *internal iliacs* are short thick trunks which soon break up into several branches to the muscles of the hind quarters. The *external iliacs*, with their continuations, are the main arteries of the hind legs. Each, as previously stated, begins below the last lumbar vertebra, curves obliquely outward and downward, giving off branches, and, near the head of the femur, receives the name of *femoral artery*.

The *femoral artery* is the artery of the thigh. Just above the back of the stifle joint it divides into two branches, the *anterior* and *posterior tibial*, the latter supplying the back part of the gaskin and hock with nourishment, while the former winds forward between the tibia and fibula to the fore part of the leg, gaining it midway between the stifle and the hock. At the hock it passes obliquely outward, crossing the joint, and becomes the *great metatarsal artery* at the upper and outer part of the metatarsus. The *great metatarsal* passes under the small splint bone and gains the back part of the cannon, then, passing down the leg, it divides just below the fork of the suspensory ligament into two branches, the *external* and *internal digitals*, which will be studied later.

The involuntary muscles of the heart receive their blood supply from two small arteries, *right* and *left coronary*, which branch off at the beginning of the common aorta.

Veins.

Veins are usually found accompanying the arteries of the body and bearing similar names; there are several important exceptions, three of which will be here noted, namely, the *anterior vena cava, jugular,* and *posterior vena cava.*

The *anterior vena cava* is the large, short vein, formed by numerous branches, returning the blood from the head, the neck, the fore leg, and part of the chest. It is located in the front part of the thorax, below the trachea, and between the right and left pleurae, and empties into the right auricle.

The *jugular veins* (right and left) are the largest branches of the anterior vena cava and collect the blood from the head and neighboring parts. Just below and back of the lower jaw they approach the carotid arteries and run down the neck in their company. Each jugular is outside of the corresponding carotid and the two are separated by a thin muscle. The jugular veins in their descent follow grooves at the side of the neck (jugular furrows), and at first are close to the surface and easily felt; they soon take a deeper course, running beneath the panniculus carnosus muscle. They enter the front part of the thorax, where they empty into the anterior vena cava just in front of the heart.

The *posterior vena cava* is the main vein returning the blood from the hind parts and from the abdominal and pelvic organs. It corresponds to the posterior aorta, which, as has been seen, is the main artery carrying the blood to these parts. This vein is formed at the front part of the pelvis and runs forward under the lumbar vertebra, accompanying the posterior aorta, which is at its left. When it reaches the upper border of the liver it inclines downward and passes through a notch or fissure of that organ. Thence it passes through the diaphragm into the thoracic cavity; here it follows a groove on the upper surface of the right lung and then enters the right auricle of the heart.

The important veins of the foot will be discussed later.

ANATOMY AND PHYSIOLOGY OF THE LYMPHATIC SYSTEM

The lymphatic or absorbent system resembles the system of blood veins with which it is connected. The main part of the system collects surplus *lymph* (to be described later) and returns it to the blood; a smaller part has the same function, but, in addition, absorbs and collects chyle and adds it to the blood.

When the blood in its circuit reaches the capillaries the *serum* oozes through their thin walls into the minute spaces in the surrounding tissues and there receives the name of *lymph*. This colorless fluid bathes and nourishes the tissues and takes up worn-out material. The spaces in the tissues assemble into minute, delicate, and transparent vessels (lymphatics), which are remarkable for their knotted appearance, due to numerous valves. The vessels join and increase in size, like veins, and through them flows the surplus lymph with its collected waste material.

The vessels of the right fore extremity, the right side of the head, neck, and thorax, form tubes uniting in a main trunk, called the *right lymphatic vein*, which leads into the anterior vena cava; the vessels from the remainder of the body unite in a trunk called the *thoracic duct*, which begins in the lumbar region, passes forward beneath the lumbar and dorsal vertebrae, and empties into the anterior vena cava, just in front of the heart.

Each of the villi of the intestines contains a minute vessel called a *lacteal*, which absorbs chyle and receives its name from the lacteal or milky appearance of that fluid. These vessels of the smaller lymphatic system unite and form larger tubes which empty into the *receptaculum chyli* (chyle reservoir), which is a part of the thoracic duct of the larger system.

It will thus be seen that the lymph with its waste material and the chyle with its nutrient material are mixed and poured into the impure blood. The lymph and chyle are taken up into the serum and the waste material is thrown off from the circulating blood by the lungs, skin, and kidneys.

Lymph, therefore, makes a circuit very much as blood does.

To simplify the explanation of the system, the lymphatic glands have not been mentioned.

Glands are organs, the function of which is to separate certain substances from the blood, which are either to be used in the animal's system or to be thrown off as waste material.

The lymphatic glands are so placed that the lymphatic vessels pass through them in their course toward the main trunks. These glands act as filters and remove any infective material from the lymph and also supply lymph corpuscles, which are identical with the white corpuscles of the blood.

When the glands are situated near diseased structures, an amount of infected material lodges in the glands, greater than can be overcome by the lymph corpuscles, and, in consequence, inflammation and swelling of the glands result.

ANATOMY OF THE NERVOUS SYSTEM

A nerve consists of a bundle of tubular fibers, held together by dense connective tissue; the nerve fibers form a conducting apparatus, to convey impulses of sensation and to transmit impulses of motion.

The nervous system is divided into two minor systems, the *cerebro-spinal*, which is to a considerable extent influenced by the will of the animal, and the *sympathetic*, which is not directly influenced by the will.

In the first the center is made up of two portions, the brain and the spinal cord.

The brain is situated in the cranial cavity; the spinal cord is elongated and continuous with the brain and is situated in the canal of the vertebral column.

The communicating portion of this system consists of the cerebro-spinal nerves, which leave the brain and spinal cord in symmetrical pairs, and are distributed to the voluntary muscles, to the organs of common sensation, and to those of special sense.

The sympathetic system consists of a double chain of *ganglia* (small brains), extending from the head to the coccyx, one chain along each side of the spine, and the two chains connected by nerve cords. The ganglia are also connected to branches of the cerebro-spinal nerves, thus uniting the two systems. The nerves of the sympathetic system are distributed to the involuntary muscles, mucous membranes, internal organs, and blood vessels.

ANATOMY OF THE EYE

The eye is the organ of sight and is situated in the orbital cavity. It is spherical in shape and is filled with fluid. The front portion, called the *cornea*, is perfectly clear and admits the light to the back part of the eye, where it strikes the *retina*, an expansion of the *optic nerve*; through this nerve impressions are conveyed to the brain. The colored portion or *iris*, situated behind the cornea, acts as a curtain, regulating the amount of light admitted through the central opening, which is called the *pupil*. The *crystalline lens* is a small transparent body situated immediately behind the pupil; it is thick in the center and tapers toward the edges. Its function is to draw the rays of light to a focus on the retina. When the lens is diseased and no light can pass through, the animal is said to have a cataract. The eyelids are two movable curtains, superior and inferior, which protect the eye. The *membrana nictitans*, or accessory eyelid (haw), is situated near the inner angle between the lids and the eyeball. This membrane acts like a finger in the removal of foreign bodies from the eye. The *conjunctiva* is a continuous mucous membrane covering the cornea and haw and lining the eyelids.

The fluid between the lens and the cornea (called *"aqueous"*) is watery, while that between the lens and the retina (called *"vitreous"*) is thicker and like the white of a raw egg.

The outer covering (seen when the animal shows the white of the eye) is a fibrous tissue called the *sclerotic coat*. Between it and the retina, is a delicate, dark colored tissue containing the blood vessels and known as the *choroid coat*.

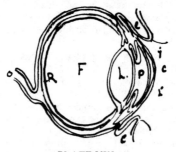

PLATE VIII

Section of the eye

c, Cornea; e, Eyelids; f, Fluid; i, Iris; l, Crystalline lens; o, Optic nerve; p, Pupil; r, Retina

26

ANATOMY OF THE SKIN

The skin consists primarily of two parts: The outer, nonvascular layer, called the *cuticle* or *epidermis*, and the deep vascular layer, called the *corium, dermis*, or true skin.

The epidermis is a scaly covering. The true skin or dermis lies immediately under the epidermis, is much thicker, and contains the roots of the hair, the sweat glands, and the *sebaceous* glands.

Sweat glands are simple tubes extending from the deeper layers of the skin to the surface of the body and pouring out perspiration, which carries with it certain waste materials from the system. The evaporation of sweat cools the body and assists in regulating its temperature.

Sebaceous glands secrete an oily fluid. On parts of the skin which are subjected to much friction these glands pour their oil directly upon the outer surface, as in the sheath, the back of the pastern joints, etc. Usually, however, the glands open into the hair follicles or sacs, and the oily secretion gives gloss to the hair, prevents it from becoming dry and brittle, and keeps the surrounding skin soft and supple.

ANATOMY AND PHYSIOLOGY OF THE FOOT

The horse's foot is composed of three parts, viz: The bony framework or skeleton, completed by certain elastic structures of cartilage and fat; the layer of highly sensitive flesh (quick), which covers the framework; and the box or case of horn, called the hoof, which incloses and protects the above-mentioned structures.

Bones of the foot.

The bones of the pastern region and foot form a column extending downward from the fetlock into the hoof, and, as previously stated, are named as follows: *Os suffraginis* (long pastern bone), *os coronae* (short pastern bone), *os pedis* (coffin bone), and *os navicularis* (shuttle bone).

The *os suffraginis* is about one-third as long as the cannon bone (the bone extending from the knee or hock to the fetlock) and reaches from the fetlock joint above to the pastern joint below; its superior extremity shows a shallow cavity on each side, separated in the middle by a deep groove, and into this surface fits the lower end of the cannon bone. The inferior extremity is much smaller and narrower than the upper; on each side is a small convex surface, the two surfaces separated in the middle by a shallow groove. This extremity meets the upper end of the os coronae and forms the pastern joint.

The *os coronae* follows the direction of the os suffraginis downward and forward and lies between the pastern and coffin joints, its lower end being within the hoof.

Its superior surface shows a shallow cavity on each side, with a ridge between them to fit the lower end of the os suffraginis. The lower surface of this bone shows a convex part on each side, separated by a groove, to fit the upper surface of the coffin bone in the coffin joint.

The *os pedis* is an irregular bone, situated within the hoof and is similar to it in shape.

The anterior surface is known as the *wall surface*; it shows a number of small openings, called *foramina*, for the passage of blood vessels and nerves, and is

27

roughened to give attachment to the soft parts *(sensitive laminae)* covering it. At the top of this surface, in front, is a ridge called the *pyramidal process*, to which is attached the extensor pedis tendon.

The lower surface, called the *sole*, is half-moon-shaped, concave and smooth, and is covered by the sensitive sole. The upper surface helps to form the coffin joint and is called the *articular surface*; it shows two shallow cavities, separated by a ridge.

Just back of the articular surface is a small triangular surface to fit the navicular bone behind.

Just back of the sole is a rough surface, to which is attached the flexor pedis perforans tendon; it is called the *tendinous surface*.

On each side of this surface is a groove running forward and terminating in an opening, called the *plantar foramen*; an artery and a nerve enter the bone and a vein leaves it through this opening.

On each side of the os pedis, extending backward, is a prolongation, called the *wing*. Each wing is divided by a notch and then by a groove, which runs forward on the outside of the bone; an artery lies in the notch and groove.

The *os navicularis* is an irregular bone situated behind and below the os coronae and behind the os pedis, articulating with both bones. Its long axis is perpendicular to the axis of the foot. The extremities of the bone are attached to the wings of the os pedis; the inferior surface is covered with cartilage, which forms a smooth surface for the movements of the tendon of the flexor pedis perforans muscle.

Elastic structures of the foot.

All of the parts of the foot, except the bones, are more or less elastic or "springy" and yield when pressure is applied; but certain parts have a very high degree of elasticity, their special use being to overcome the effects of concussion or jar when the foot strikes the ground and to prevent injury, and these parts are referred to as the elastic structures of the foot. They are the *lateral cartilages* and *plantar cushion*, or fatty frog, as it is sometimes called.

The *lateral cartilages* are thin plates of cartilage, one attached to the top of each wing of the os pedis, and extending backward and upward so far that their upper borders may be felt under the skin above the coronet at the heels.

The *plantar cushion* is a very elastic wedge-shaped pad, which fills up the space between the two lateral cartilages on the sides, the sensitive frog below, and the flexor pedis perforans tendon above.

The point or anterior part of the plantar cushion extends forward to the ridge which separates the sole from the tendinous surface of the os pedis. The base is covered by the skin above the heels.

Sensitive structures of the foot.

Over the bones and elastic structures of the foot is found a complete covering of very sensitive flesh, and from each part of this covering some part of the hoof is secreted or formed. The divisions of this layer of flesh are called the sensitive parts or structures of the foot. They are the *coronary band, sensitive laminae, sensitive sole, sensitive frog*, and the *coronary frog band*.

The *coronary band* is a thick convex band of tough flesh, about four-fifths of an inch wide, and extends entirely around the top of the hoof from one bulb of the heel to the other; in front it is attached to the extensor pedis tendon, and on the sides to ligaments of the coffin joint, to the lower end of the os coronae, and to the

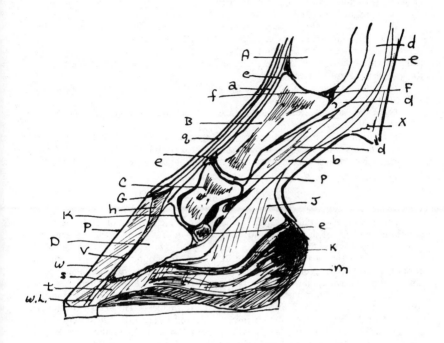

PLATE IX

Parts of the hoof and pastern.

A.	Cannon bone	f.	Articular cartilage
B.	Os suffraginis	g.	Perioplic ring
C.	Os coronae	h.	Coronary band
D.	Os pedis	j.	Plantar cushion
E.	Os navicularis	k.	Sensitive frog
F.	Fetlock joint	m.	Horny frog
K.	Coffin Joint	p.	Periople
P.	Pastern joint	q.	Skin
a.	Extensor pedis tendon	s.	Senstive sole
b.	Flexor pedis perforans tendon	t.	Horny sole
c.	Flexor pedis perforatus tendon	v.	Sensitive laminae
d.	Sesamoidian ligaments	w.l.	White line
e.	Capsular ligament	x.	Ergot

29

lateral cartilages. The surface of the coronary band is covered with small pointed projections or villi. The coronary band secretes or forms the principal part (middle layer) of the wall of the hoof.

The *sensitive laminae* (fleshy leaves) cover and are firmly attached to the anterior or wall surface of the os pedis and to the lower part of the outer surface of the lateral cartilages. These delicate leaves of the flesh dovetail into the horny laminae which they secrete and, with them, serve to fasten the wall of the hoof to the os pedis and to the lateral cartilages.

The *sensitive sole* covers the sole surface of the os pedis, is covered with villi, and secretes the horny sole.

The *sensitive frog* covers the lower face of the plantar cushion, and from its villi the horny frog is secreted.

The *coronary frog band* or *perioplic ring* is a narrow band of flesh running around just above the coronary band and separated from it by a faint groove. From the fine villi on the surface of this ring the delicate fibers grow which form the *periople*.

The hoof.

The box or case of horn, called the hoof, which incloses and protects the other structures of the foot, is divided into three parts – *wall, sole,* and *frog.* In a healthy foot these parts are solidly united.

The *wall* is the part seen when the foot is on the ground; it extends from the edge of the hair to the ground and is divided into the *toe, quarters, heels,* and *bars*; it has an internal surface, an external surface, and an upper and lower border.

The *toe* is the front part of the wall. It is steeper in the hind foot than in the fore. The *quarters* extend backward from the toe to the heels. The *heel* or buttress is that part of the wall where it bends inward and forward, and the *bar* is the division of the wall running from the heel to within about 1 inch of the point or apex of the frog. It lies between the horny sole and the frog.

The external surface of the wall is covered by a thin varnish-like coat of fine horn, called the *periople.*

The internal surface of the wall is covered by from 500 to 600 thin plates of leaves of horn, called the *horny laminae.* Between the horny laminae, which run parallel to each other and in a direction downward and forward, there are fissures into which dovetail the sensitive laminae, and this union, as previously stated, binds the wall of the hoof to the os pedis and lateral cartilages.

The upper border of the wall shows a deep groove (coronary groove) into which fits the coronary band.

The lower border is called the "bearing edge" (or "spread" in the unshod foot) and is the part to which the shoe is fitted.

The *horny sole* is a thick plate of horn, somewhat half-moon-shaped, and has two surfaces and two borders.

The upper surface is convex (round or bulging upward) and is in union with the sensitive sole from which the horny sole grows. The lower surface is concave or hollowed out and is covered with scales or crusts of dead horn, which gradually loosen and fall off.

The outer border of the sole joins the inner part of the lower border of the wall by means of a ring of soft horn, called the *white line.* This mark or line is sometimes called the *guide line,* as it shows where the nail should be started in shoeing.

30

The inner border is a V-shaped notch and is in union with the bars, except at its narrow part where it joins the frog.

The horny sole protects the sensitive sole and does not, in a healthy foot, bear weight, except a very narrow border at the white line, an eighth or tenth of an inch in width.

The *horny frog* is the wedge-shaped mass of horn filling up the triangular space between the bars. The lower face shows two prominent ridges, separated behind by a cavity, called the *cleft*, and joining in front at the *apex* or point of the frog; these ridges terminate behind in the bulbs of the frog. Between the sides of the frog and the bars are two cavities, called the *commissures*. The upper surface of the horny frog is the exact reverse of the lower and shows in the middle of a ridge of horn, called the *frog stay*, which assists in forming a firm union between the horny and sensitive frog. The horny frog serves to break the jar or concussion by acting as a cushion or pad; it protects the sensitive frog and prevents the foot from slipping.

Structure of horn.

The horn of the hoof presents a fibrous appearance and consists of very fine horn fibers or tubes, similar to hairs, running downward and forward and held together by a cementing substance. The horn fibers of wall, sole, and frog all run in the same direction, downward and forward, the only difference being that those of the frog are much finer and softer and run in wavy lines, whereas the fibers of wall and sole are straight.

The horn fibers grow from the small villi, which cover the surfaces of the coronary band, sensitive sole, and sensitive frog.

Circulation of blood through the foot.

In previous study of the arteries we have seen that the large *metacarpal* of the fore leg and the *great metatarsal* of the hind leg each divides just above the fetlock into two branches. These branches are called the *external* and *internal digital* arteries, one on the inner and one on the outer side of the fetlock joint. They follow the borders of the flexor tendons downward and terminate inside of the wings of the os pedis. Each of the internal and external digital arteries gives off five branches – the *perpendicular, transverse, artery of the frog, preplantar ungual,* and *plantar ungual.*

The *perpendicular artery* is given off at right angles about the middle of the os suffraginis, descends on the side of the pastern, bends forward and joins with the artery of the same name from the opposite side ad forms the *superficial coronary arch*. From this arch branches descend to the coronary band.

The *transverse artery* comes off under the upper border of the lateral cartilage, runs forward, and joins its fellow from the opposite side between the extensor pedis tendon and the os coronae. The *deep coronary arch* is the name given to this arrangement of the arteries, and branches from this arch also supply the coronary band.

The *artery of the frog* rises behind the pastern joint at the upper border of the lateral cartilage. It has two branches – a posterior, which runs back and supplies the bulb of the heel, and an anterior, which runs forward and downward through the plantar cushion and supplies the sensitive frog.

The *preplantar ungual artery* is given off inside the wing of the os pedis, passes through the preplantar notch, and runs forward along the preplantar groove on the side of the bone. It helps supply the sensitive laminae with blood and sends some small branches into the bone to join branches from other arteries.

The *plantar ungual artery* is the terminal or last branch of the digital artery (is a continuation of that artery) and enters the os pedis at the plantar foramen.

The two plantar ungual arteries run forward within the bone and unite to form the *circulus arteriosus*. From this circle spring ascending and descending branches. The ascending branches, called the *anterior laminal* arteries, leave the bone through the small openings (foramina) and supply the sensitive laminae in front. The descending branches, called the *inferior communicating* arteries, are about fourteen in number and emerge from the bone by the openings just above its lower edge; they unite to form a large trunk, running around the toe of the os pedis, called the *circumflex* artery, and this artery gives off ascending and descending branches. The ascending branches pass into the sensitive laminae, and the descending branches, called the *solar* arteries, numbering about fourteen, run backward through the sensitive sole to form a second circle, called the *inferior circumflex* artery.

The *veins* of the foot are arranged in networks, each network or plexus named from the parts in which it is located. The solar plexus is found running all through the sensitive sole. The laminal plexus runs through and under the sensitive laminae. The coronary plexus surrounds the os coronae and upper part of the os pedis, just under the coronary band.

The veins of the frog are those found in the plantar cushion and sensitive frog; the interosseous veins form a network within the os pedis. The veins of the foot all unite above to form a large trunk, called the digital vein, which runs along the digital artery and carries the blood back toward the heart. The veins of the foot are valveless below the middle of the pastern, an arrangement which allows the blood to flow in either direction when pressure is applied and thus prevents injury.

Nerves of the foot.

The nerves of the foot supply feeling or the sense of touch to the parts. The large nerve cord on either side of the limb divides at the fetlock joint into three branches, called the digital nerves – the anterior, the posterior, and the middle.

The anterior digital nerve passes downward and forward and supplies the anterior or front part of the foot.

The posterior digital nerve, the largest of the three, passes down behind the digital artery to supply the structures in the posterior part of the foot. It gives off a branch which passes through the notch in the wing of the os pedis (in company with the preplantar ungual artery) to supply some of the sensitive laminae; it also sends branches into the os pedis with the plantar ungual artery.

The middle branch is very small, is said to always join the anterior branch, and supplies the sensitive sole and fetlock pad.

The functions of most of the parts of the foot have been mentioned in passing, but there are some points in connection with the physiology of the foot which need to be explained more in detail.

Expansion and contraction.

When weight comes upon the leg, the os pedis descends slightly and causes the sole to descend and flatten. The plantar cushion and horny frog are compressed between the ground below and the structures above; this compression causes them to spread out sidewise, carrying outward the lateral cartilages and bars and the wall at the quarters. This is called *expansion*. When weight is removed from the leg, the plantar cushion becomes thicker and narrower, and the lateral cartilages and quarters move inward to where they were before expanding. This is called *contraction*. The elastic lateral cartilage is merely a flexible extension of the wing of the os pedis and would appear to have been specially designed for expansion and contraction at the quarters. It is also to be noted that the bars are a provision for this same purpose, since expansion and contraction could not take place if the wall formed a solid unbroken ring around the hoof.

In addition to breaking the jar when the foot comes to the ground, the plantar cushion has another important use. It assists in the circulation of the blood through the veins of the foot. When weight is placed upon the foot the pressure on the plantar cushion forces the blood upward through the veins; then, when the foot is lifted and the pressure is removed from the horny frog and plantar cushion, the veins of the frog again fill with blood, and this pumping action is repeated with each step. Proof of this statement is seen when a digital vein is cut, by accident or in experiment. If the horse is walked, a jet of blood spurts out each time he puts the foot to the ground; but if he is allowed to stand the blood flows in a steady stream from the vein. Great injury to the foot results from starting the horse off suddenly at a fast gait on a hard road after he has been standing for some time or when he first comes out of the stable. The circulation (just explained) and the structures of the foot should have time to gradually adapt themselves to the change from rest to severe work.

Moisture.

The wall of the healthy hoof is, by weight, about one-fourth water, the sole more than one-third, and the frog almost one-half. This water is supplied by the blood and preserves the horn in a tough and elastic condition. The hoof, particularly the frog, is capable of absorbing moisture from the ground. The periople, which covers the wall, prevents the evaporation of water, and therefore should *never* be rasped. As there is no similar covering for the sole and the frog, the layers of horn on their exposed surfaces dry out and die. The dead layers are hard and brittle, and gradually fall or flake off; but, as they preserve the moisture in the layers of live horn beneath, they should not be removed in preparing the hoof for shoeing.

Shoeing.

Shoeing is a necessary evil, but by remembering the functions of the various parts of the foot the damage resulting may be limited to a comparatively small amount.

The following rules may serve as a guide for the shoeing of healthy feet:

1.   The wall, being the weight bearer, should be rasped perfectly level or the foot will be thrown out of its true position, causing extra strain on some of the ligaments.

2.   Fit the shoe accurately to the outline of the foot; do not alter the latter to fit the shoe. Rasping away the exterior of the crust to fit the shoe not only renders the horn brittle but is so much loss of bearing surface.

3.   The sole should not be touched with the knife; loose flakes may be removed with a blunt instrument.

4.   The bars should not be cut away; they are a part of the wall and intended to carry weight. The shoe should rest on them.

5.   The frog should not be cut, but left to attain its full growth. No frog can perform its functions unless on a level with the ground surface of the shoe.

6.   The shoe should have a true and level bearing and rest well and firmly on the wall and bars.

A plain light-weight shoe is the best – plain on both ground and foot surface.

7.   High nailing is injurious; do not use any more nails than are absolutely necessary, as the nails destroy the horn.

CHAPTER IV

ADMINISTRATION OF MEDICINES – WEIGHTS AND MEASURES

ADMINISTRATION OF MEDICINES

Medicines may enter the body through any of the following designated channels: First, by the mouth; second, by the lungs and upper air passages; third, by the skin; fourth, under the skin (hypodermically); fifth, by the rectum; and sixth, by intravenous injection.

By the mouth. Medicines can be given by the mouth in the form of powders, balls, and drenches.

By the air passages. Medicines are administered to the lungs and upper air passages by inhalations and nasal douches.

By the skin. Care must be taken in applying some medicines over too large a portion of the body at any one time, as poisoning and death may follow from too rapid absorption through the skin. For domestic animals medicines are to be applied to the skin for local purposes or diseases only.

By the rectum. Medicines may be given by the rectum when we can not give or have them retained by the mouth; when we want local action; to destroy the small worms infesting the large bowels; to stimulate the natural movement of the intestine and cause an evacuation; and to nourish the body.

WEIGHTS AND MEASURES

Solid measure.[a]

60 grains (gr.) . . . . 1 dram (   ).
8 drams . . . . .1 ounce (   ).
16 ounces . . . . 1 pound (lb.).

Liquid measure.

60 minims (min.) . . . . 1 fluid dram (f.   ).
8 fluid drams . . . . 1 fluid ounce (f.   ).
16 fluid ounces . . . . .1 pint (O.).
32 fluid ounces . . . . 1 quart (Oii.).
4 quarts . . . . 1 gallon (Ci.).

PRESCRIPTIONS

In writing prescriptions, Roman numerals are used instead of Arabic (ordinary figures) and the numerals follow the symbols, thus: vii for 7 drams; f xii for 12 fluid drams, etc. S. S. signifies one half, thus: ii s.s. for 2½ drams.

[a]The difference in weight between the apothecaries' ounce (480 grains) and the ounce avoirdupois (437.5 grains) is neglected in handling veterinary or bulky medicines.

FIELD EXPEDIENTS

In stables, doses must be accurately measured by scales or graduates, according to the tables of dry or liquid measure, but in the field the following *rough* expedients may be used:

Dry measure.

1 ounce of lead acetate

A large spoon. . . . .
Heaping full.)

1 ounce of a salt

Tin cup . . . . 7/8 of a quart.
Full day's ration of medium-weight oats.   14 cups.

Liquid measure.

A drop . . . . 1 minim.
A teaspoonful . . . . .1 fluid dram.
A tablespoonful . . . . 1/2 fluid ounce.
Tin cup . . . . 28 ounces=7/8 of a quart.

CHAPTER V

WOUNDS, SPRAINS, BRUISES, ABRASIONS, AND ABSCESSES

Wounds and Their Treatment.

Wounds (separations of the soft tissues) are classed as: *Incised wounds*, or cuts; *lacerated wounds*, or tears; and *punctured wounds*, or holes.

A *dressing* is a local, periodically repeated treatment, producing a continued action, and often following the performance of an operation. It is the application upon the surface of the wound of healing substances, which, in some cases, are mechanically held in place by bandages, stitches, etc.

Before applying a dressing the wound should be thoroughly cleansed and freed from blood, pus, the remains of previous dressing, and, in a word, of any foreign or other substances capable of becoming sources of irritation. This is best done with water, but the effect is frequently greatly improved by combining with it some of the antiseptics, such as carbolic acid, creolin, bichloride of mercury, etc.

Antiseptics are remedies which prevent putrefaction, or rotting, and their combinations with water are called *solutions*.

The solution may be applied by carefully passing a saturated ball of oakum over the surface of the wound, or it may be used more freely in larger ablutions (washing). Crusts or scabs, if present, may be removed with the scissors or scraped away with the knife, but the finger nails must never be used for such a purpose, for the practice is both filthy and dangerous. The wound is to be handled only when necessary; all needless handling irritates. If the wound is deep, it should be cleansed by syringing.

The essential condition of cleanliness applies not only to the wound but also to the materials used for dressings, and soiled cloths or bandages and dirty oakum must be rigorously rejected; everything coming in contact with a wound must be absolutely clean, hands as well as instruments and dressings. Instruments, however, should never be immersed in the bichloride solution, which rapidly corrodes metal.

In the treatment of all wounds cleanliness is of more importance than medication, but the two in combination, when thoroughly and intelligently carried out, will leave no room for the propagation and ravages of those germs that cause the formation of pus and retard the healing process. The farrier, or the man who is to care for the injured animal, should have his hands thoroughly clean, and should procure in a clean can or bucket a solution of creolin or other antiseptic, and several clean pieces of cotton, gauze, or oakum. Sponges are cleaned with difficulty and should not be used.

If hemorrhage (bleeding) is profuse the first step is to arrest the flow of blood by ligating (tying) the blood vessel or vessels with a piece of silk, or if none is at hand, with a clean piece of string; if the blood vessels can not be tied, a thick pad made of cotton or of several layers of gauze or clean cloth, folded so as to cover the wound, and held firmly in place by one or more cotton bandages, will check the flow of blood. This arrangement, called a *compress*, should be left on until the hemorrhage ceases, and the wound treated as described later.

In applying dressings (except compresses) unnecessary pressure should be avoided, especially on the soft tissues.

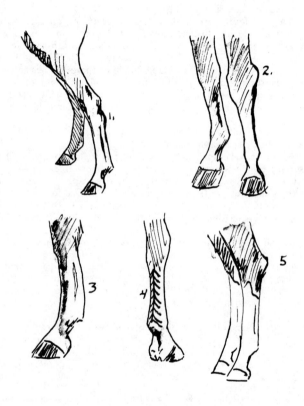

PLATE X

Fig. 1, Curb. Fig. 2, Bursal Enlargement. Fig. 3, Sprain of the Flexor Tendons (Bowed Tendons). Fig. 4, Line Firing. Fig. 5, Capped Hock.

Incised wounds. If the injury is one that can be sutured (sewed) a needle and silk should be immersed in a solution of creolin – creolin 1 part, water 50 parts; the hair around the wound should either be shaved or be clipped with a pair of shears, and the wound thoroughly cleansed by washing it with cotton saturated with the creolin solution; all dirt and hair must be removed, all ragged edges, if any, cut away and the edges of the wound placed in contact with each other if possible and held in place by the aid of sutures, care being taken to allow free drainage; the wound should then be wiped dry with a fresh piece of cotton or gauze, and over the surface should be dusted some iodoform or acetanilid. If the location will permit, the wound should be covered with a pad of gauze or absorbent cotton, and a cotton bandage wrapped around the parts to hold the pad in place. The wound should be dressed once or twice a day until the formation of pus ceases; when the wound is dry, only the powder should be used.

Lacerated wounds. If the wound is a large one, with the skin and tissues so badly torn and lacerated as not to admit of the use of sutures, the torn and ragged edges (especially if the lower part of the wound hangs down) should be removed with the knife or scissors and the wound dressed as above directed. When the wound begins to granulate (fill with new tissue) care should be taken that the granulations are not allowed to grow out higher than the skin, causing the condition known as *proud flesh.*

The treatment of proud flesh consists in the removal of the unhealthy tissue by the use of the knife or by the application of a red-hot iron; burnt alum or salicylic acid dusted upon the surface of the wound will destroy the unhealthy granules.

Punctured wounds. Punctured wounds (except those around joints) should be explored with a probe to ascertain if any foreign bodies are in the channel; if so, they should be removed, and if necessary a dependent opening be made to allow perfect drainage. The parts should then be syringed out thoroughly with a solution of creolin, 1 to 50; carbolic acid, 1 to 20 or 30; or bichloride of mercury, 1 to 1,000, and the outside opening sprinkled with iodoform. This treatment should be applied twice daily.

For a few days the wound should be swabbed with tincture of iodine or packed with strips of gauze saturated with this drug in order to destroy infection, check the formation of pus, and promote the growth of healthy tissue.

Wounds of the lips, nostrils, and eyelids heal very rapidly; if of several days' standing, they should have their edges scraped and then be sutured, and iodoform or acetanilid dusted over the surface twice daily.

An excellent antiseptic solution for the treatment of wounds during fly time is made by dissolving 8 ounces of gum camphor in 3 ounces of carbolic acid. Apply with a clean swab several times daily. One ounce of creolin to 8 ounces of olive oil is a good substitute.

Punctured wounds around joints.

Open joint is a wound situated on a joint and extending through the capsular ligament, allowing the joint oil to escape.

Treatment. Remove the hair and thoroughly clean the parts around the wound with a solution of bichloride of mercury, 1 to 1,000; unless a foreign body is known to be lodged in it, do not probe or explore, as the introduction of any instrument, even if thoroughly clean, will be the means of setting up considerable inflammation. Apply a blister of biniodide of mercury 1 part, cosmoline 4 parts, for the purpose of closing the opening, limiting motion, and relieving pain. Use the slings if the wound is very painful. If the wound is so large that a blister will not close it, the treatment should be as prescribed for an open wound.

A punctured tendon sheath is treated like a punctured joint.

CAUSE AND TREATMENT OF SPRAINS

Sprains affect muscles, tendons, and ligaments. The fibers of which they are composed are severely stretched, sometimes torn in serious cases, causing inflammation and subsequent contraction, and, in case of muscles, atrophy or sweeny (wasting away).

Strains of the muscles.

Muscle strains occur in various parts of the trunk and limbs; thus, a horse may strain the neck muscles, as a result of falling on the head; the muscles of the dorsal region may be strained by the hind feet slipping backward. When a muscle is strained the injury is succeeded by pain, swelling heat, and loss of function.

An inflamed muscle can no longer contract; hence in some strains the symptoms resemble those of paralysis.

Sprains of the suspensory ligament and flexor tendons.
("Breakdown" and "Bowed tendons")

The fibrous structures situated behind the cannon bone, both in the front and hind legs, are often the seat of lacerations or sprains resulting from violent efforts or sudden jerks. The injury is easily recognized by the changed appearance of the parts, which become more or less swollen; the swelling usually extending from the knee down to the fetlock and occasionally even farther. It is always characterized by heat and is variously sensitive, ranging from a mere tenderness to a degree of soreness which shrinks from the lightest touch. The degree of lameness corresponds to the severity of the injury.

Sprains of ligaments.

The calcaneo-cuboid ligament, situated at the back part of the hock and uniting the calcaneum, the cuboid, and the external splint bones, is frequently sprained. This condition is known as a "curb."

The various ligaments entering into the formation of joints are subject to sprains and injuries. This condition is indicated by lameness, accompanied by pain, heat, and swelling.

The capsular ligament when sprained very often becomes weakened, resulting in distention of the synovial sac. Bursal enlargements receive different names, according to their location. *Bog spavin* is a characteristic bursal enlargement. It is found on the front and inner side of the hock joint and varies in size with the amount of distention of the capsular ligament. The trouble is usually caused by slipping, hard and fast work, irregular exercise, and high feeding. Draft animals, pulling heavy loads over rough or slippery ground, are particularly subject to this injury, which is also more commonly seen in young than in mature animals. The swelling can be readily detected; under pressure it fluctuates; heat may or may not be present; lameness rarely results unless the injury be accompanied by complications, such as *bone spavin* or bony deposits.

40

In sprain of the stifle joint, the ligaments holding it in position are severely stretched, in some cases sprained or ruptured, and even dislocation of the patella may occur. In this trouble the patella is forced outward and thus makes the joint immovable, the leg being extended backward and the foot resting on the toe. If the animal is forced to move, he drags the leg, being unable to bring it forward in the natural manner on account of the dislocation. The bone is returned to place in the following manner: A rope having been placed about the pastern, the leg is steadily drawn forward by one or more assistants, while the operator stretches the patella forward and inward. When the bone regains its proper position, the animal has proper control of his leg. Reduce the inflammation promptly and blister as explained below. In case the patella persists in slipping out again, a rope should be fastened to the pastern and attached to the collar about the horse's neck; the rope should be drawn tight enough to prevent the horse extending his leg to the rear, but allowing him to stand upon it; keep the rope on until the blister has worked.

General treatment of sprains. Perfect rest is absolutely necessary and must never be overlooked in the treatment of all sprains; therefore the injured animal should be at once removed to a level stall where it can remain until complete recovery has taken place. Hot or cold applications should be applied to the injured parts. These applications should be in the form of fomentations (bathing), or bandages saturated with water. Flannel bandages must not be allowed to dry while in contact with the injured parts, as flannel applied wet, shrinks in drying, and will not only retard the reparative process, but cause unnecessary pain. Cold water is often materially assisted in accomplishing the desired results by the addition of acetate of lead or sulphate of zinc, witch-hazel, or nitrate of potash. A convenient solution is made as follows: Acetate of lead and sulphate of zinc, each 1 ounce; water, 1 quart; or, 1 pint of witch-hazel, 1 ounce of acetate of lead, and water enough to make 1 quart. If pain is very severe the following may be used: Tincture opium, 4 ounces; acetate of lead, 2 ounces; water to make 1 quart; this application is of more benefit when applied warm. All applications should be used several times daily.

If, after the inflammation is reduced, the parts remain large and swollen, benefit will result from the application of tincture of iodine, well rubbed in, twice a day. If this treatment fails to restore the parts to their normal condition in a reasonable length of time, a blister should be applied. It is made as follows: Cantharides (powdered) 1 part, cosmoline 4 to 5 parts; or, cantharides (powdered) 1 part, biniodide mercury 1 part, cosmoline 4 to 6 parts.

Before applying either the blister or the iodine the hair should be clipped from the parts to which the medicine is to be applied. To obtain the best results from the blister it should be well rubbed in for at least fifteen minutes. The animal must be tied in such a manner that he can not reach the blistered part with his mouth; the blister should be left on for a period of twenty-four to forty-eight hours; it must then be removed by washing with warm water and castile soap. After the blister has been removed the animal may be untied. The parts should be kept clean, free from scabs, and soft from the use of cosmoline, olive oil, or glycerin.

Rest is necessary throughout the treatment, and even to test his soundness the animal should not be moved more than is necessary.

If the disease does not yield to blisters, the parts must be fired. For this operation, two kinds of instruments are used: The *thermocautery*, which generates its own heat, and the more common form, the iron heated in the fire. Two methods of firing are in general use: *Line firing*, for diseases of the tendons, ligaments, etc., and *puncture firing*, for diseases of the bone.

BRUISES

In the riding horse the most frequent bruises are saddle and cinch galls, and bruises of the withers.

Certain horses suffer more than others, on account of the presence of old sores, scars, or scabs, or because of peculiarities in conformation.

The principal defects in conformation (previously noted) are: Abnormally high or abnormally low and thick withers; the keel-shaped breast, accompanied by flat ribs and light flanks, and the broad or bulging barrel.

Old horses sometimes have the muscles in the saddle bed atrophied, and are therefore more liable to contract saddle galls.

All horses, whatever their conformation, are subject to saddle and cinch galls, produced mechanically by three causes: First, unequal distribution of weight; second, faults in saddling and cinching; third, poor riding.

After a long ride, the blood vessels under the saddle and cinch are compressed and almost empty. If it is suspected that saddle or cinch galls may have been formed, it is advisable to leave the saddle on for a half hour to an hour after dismounting; the cinch should be loosened *very slightly*.

If pressure be suddenly and completely removed, blood is vigorously forced into the paralyzed vessels, and may rupture their walls. On the other hand, if the saddle is allowed to remain some time in position, circulation is gradually restored without injury.

Treatment. As soon as a swelling is noticed, application of cold in the form of pads kept saturated with cold water and massage in the form of gentle stroking with the fingers will aid in the absorption of the fluids causing the swelling.

Injuries to the withers require different treatment — cold applications without pressure and without massage, on account of the danger of the fluids burrowing.

A solution made of the following is a very good application for bruises: Sugar of lead 2 ounces, laudanum 4 ounces, water to make 1 quart. To be applied several times daily. Or a poultice made of flaxseed meal, to which has been added an antiseptic, such as creolin, carbolic acid, etc.

Bruises caused by kicks or running against an obstacle should be treated by applications of water, and if painful, an anodyne (pain reducing) liniment. The following makes a good anodyne: Witch-hazel 2 parts, tincture opium 1 part, tincture aconite ¼part, water 2 parts. Apply locally with the hand.

Harness horses are subject to the same injuries, produced by the saddle and cinch, as are riding horses, and, in addition, may be bruised about the neck and shoulders by the collar. If the collar has not broken or chafed the skin (see "Abrasions") treat the bruises as previously directed.

The *white lotion*, composed of 1 ounce each of sugar of lead and sulphate of zinc, water 1 quart, is a most excellent remedy for bruises and also for abrasions.

Bruises of the sole and heel.

These are quite frequent, and should be treated by hot or cold applications, accomplished by holding the foot in a tub or pail of water, or by incasing the foot in a hot flaxseed-meal poultice. If pus forms, the underrun horn must be removed and the parts kept clean and covered.

Capped elbow — shoe boil.

.This is a bruise at the point of the elbow, and is caused by the horse lying on the heels of his shoe; to prevent further injury, place a large roll around the pastern at night, and apply tincture of iodine twice daily, until the swelling is removed. In case of great swelling and heat, apply hot and cold water, or the white lotion, until the heat disappears; then proceed as above.

Capped hock.

Capped hock is a swelling, more or less soft, found on the point of the hock, and usually caused by kicking in the stall, or by bruising the parts during transportation by rail or sea. Tincture of iodine is a very good remedy for this injury.

Only in extreme cases is it advisable to use the knife in the treatment of shoe boils and capped hock. As soon as the parts are opened pus rapidly forms, and the inflammation (infection by germs) may extend to the inner structures, causing a condition that will not readily yield to treatment.

Sitfast.

Sitfasts are patches of dry, dead skin, and may involve the deeper tissues; they are caused by continuous pressure of the saddle, cinch, or collar, and may be situated on the side of the body, back, side of withers, shoulder or neck.

Treatment. With the knife remove all dead and bruised tissue, stimulate the sore at the sides by the use of lunar caustic, and treat as a common wound. When there is no more formation of pus, and the parts are perfectly dry, do not apply liquids, but use iodoform until well.

Fistulous withers.

Fistulous withers is an abscess (gathering) having a more or less chronic discharge of pus from one or more openings situated in the immediate vicinity of the withers; it may involve only the soft structures, or the bones may also be affected; it is caused by a bruise, and generally, in the army, by a bruise from an ill-fitting saddle.

Treatment. Treat as explained under "Abscesses." If, after a reasonable length of time, results are not satisfactory, a surgical operation is necessary.

Poll evil.

Poll evil is the result of a bruise on the poll. It is similar to fistulous withers, and should receive the same treatment.

ABRASIONS

An abrasion, or chafe, is an inflammation of the skin, resulting from friction. Parts of the equipment frequently wear away the hair and leave the skin raw and tender.

Treatment. One ounce of tannic acid in a pint of witchhazel is especially valuable for collar chafes; zinc oxide as a dusting powder is effective, and the white lotion is always beneficial. In emergencies, bathe the parts with cold water to which a little salt has been added.

Rope burn.

Rope burn is an abrasion, usually at the back of the pastern, and caused by the animal becoming entangled in the halter shank, picket line, or lariat. The injury may be simply a chafe of the superficial layer of the skin or it may involve the deeper structures. In the latter case it is of a serious nature and requires careful attention.

Treatment. If possible, give the animal complete rest. Clip the hair from the injured parts, at the same time removing any torn skin; wash with some good antiseptic, such as solution of creolin or carbolic acid, and apply a dusting powder, such as zinc oxide or iodoform, the former preferably. Apply a pad of clean cotton and secure with a cotton bandage; change the dressing daily. Should the parts be slow in healing, an occasional dressing of tincture of iodine is beneficial, and good results are often obtained by alternating this with a dressing of olive oil 3 parts and creolin 2 parts. Should proud flesh appear, the three sulphates (iron, copper, and zinc) may be used, or powdered copper sulphate alone. Use until the granules disappear. When the wound begins to heal nicely, it is better to dispense with the pad and bandage.

ABSCESSES

An abscess is an unnatural collection, in the tissues, of fluids, such as pus or serum. It is the result of inflammation caused by an injury or by the infection of pus germs. The swelling usually softens at some point, unless it be filled with serum, in which case it is soft and fluctuates at all points, and lies directly beneath the skin.

Soft, puffy swellings in the neighborhood of joints and tendons should not be mistaken for abscesses, as they are usually bursal enlargements, filled with synovia, and requiring different treatment. (See "General treatment of sprains.")

Treatment. A pus abscess, if slow in development, should be poulticed until it softens at some part where it can be opened by cutting through the skin; then insert a blunt instrument through the wall into the pus cavity, thus avoiding any danger of injury to blood vessels or other structures. When freely opened, the cavity should be flushed out twice daily with some antiseptic solution, care being exercised to prevent the external wound from healing before the formation of the pus has ceased. In every case provision must be made for free drainage at the lowest point.

A serious abscess (one in which we find the yellowish, watery, and often bloody serum) is treated as follows: Clip the hair away and wash the skin with an antiseptic; with an instrument that has been thoroughly disinfected make a small opening; after all fluid has escaped apply a blister of biniodide of mercury, 1 to 6, over the outside of the area occupied by the original swelling. If it fills again, repeat the treatment.

Soft, puffy swellings on the abdominal wall must be carefully examined. They may be the results of rupture, in which case opening would be fatal.

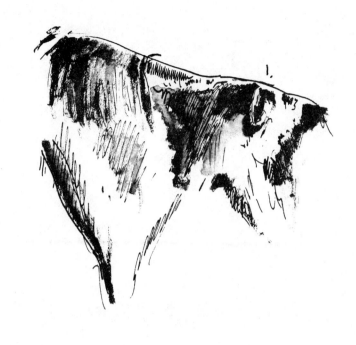

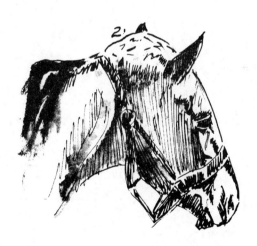

PLATE XI

Fig. 1, Fistulous withers. Fig. 2, Poll evil.

45

CHAPTER VI

DISEASES OF THE RESPIRATORY SYSTEM AND INFLUENZA

Acute Nasal Catarrh.

Acute nasal catarrh (simple cold in the head) is usually caused by standing in a draft, and may be detected by the discharge from the nostrils. It is usually accompanied by a cough, loss of appetite, and elevation of temperature (fever). The discharge is at first of the consistency of water, but may in severe cases become much thicker, and form dry crusts on the edges of the nostrils.

Treatment. The mild form does not require treatment; it ends rapidly in a cure. In severe cases, the animal should have complete rest; fumigation (steaming) from a hot solution of creolin or carbolic acid (1 ounce to ½ pail of hot water) constitutes an excellent local treatment. Give bran mashes, and administer twice daily ½ ounce of saltpeter, or 2 drams of chloride of ammonia, until the animal has recovered; the chloride of ammonia is best administered on the tongue. If the cough is frequent and the horse has difficulty in swallowing, the following liniment should be applied to the throat: Solution of ammonia 1 part, oil of turpentine 1 part, olive oil 2 parts. Apply twice daily.

Chronic Nasal Catarrh.

Chronic nasal catarrh is usually an unfavorable termination of simple catarrh; or it may result from injury and chronic inflammation of the nasal cavities; from tumors, parasites, abscesses, etc., in the nasal cavities; from diseases of the teeth; from chronic diseases of the respiratory (breathing) apparatus in general; and from chronic constitutional diseases.

Symptoms. The discharge is quite thick and becomes glued to the sides of the nostrils; its color varies from a dirty white to a yellowish gray; it frequently has a fetid (foul) odor; the quantity varies; the discharge is usually from one nostril, but both may be affected; in cases of long standing small ulcers (sores) may occasionally be seen in the nostrils; they are superficial (on the surface), are defined by sharp edges that are not thickened, and heal without leaving a scar. (The ulcer of glanders, which will be studied later, has edges shaped like saw teeth, and when healed leaves a jagged scar.)

Treatment. Is usually local and as follows: Fumigation with hot water, to which antiseptics have been added (2 ounces of creolin or 2 ounces of carbolic acid to a half bucketful of water); the steaming to continue at least one-half hour twice daily. If no definite cause of the discharge can be found, good results may be obtained by administering 2 drams of powdered copper sulphate or the same amount of iron sulphate, in the food or in a ball, once daily. In most cases, when the discharge is from one nostril only, an operation is necessary to effect a cure.

As the symptoms of this disease are so similar to glanders, the animal should be isolated, and the utensils, such as buckets, forks, brooms, currycombs, blankets, etc., should not be used about other horses, until by the use of mallein (see Glanders) the disease has been definitely determined.

Pharyngitis and Laryngitis — Sore Throat.

Sore throat is an inflammation of the lining membrane immediately in the rear of the mouth and is caused by irritating medicines, by bodies bruising the tissues, by sudden changes in the temperature, and by infection.

Symptoms. Diminution of the appetite, cough, stiffness of the head, soreness when pressure is applied to the throat, a considerable amount of mucus and saliva in the mouth, escaping in long, transparent threads, and usually a profuse thick discharge from the nose. Swallowing of liquids is painful; they are ejected through the nose, and are often of a greenish color and contain quantities of food. Temperature may range from normal to 106° F., with difficulty in breathing.

Treatment. The sick animal should be separated from the healthy ones and placed in a comfortable box stall, free from drafts, but well ventilated, and should be given green food or very fine hay, steamed oats, bran, or gruel; fresh water should be left within reach. Four drams of either ammonium chloride or potassium nitrate should be added to the drinking water.

The lips and nostrils should be kept perfectly clean and the mouth washed frequently with fresh water. Cold compresses should be used if the parts are hot, tender, and painful. In a mild case, use the ammonia liniment as in acute nasal catarrh. If an abscess is likely to form, poultices of linseed meal may be applied, and the abscess, when ready, should be opened, but never with a knife. Cut through the skin only and then insert a blunt instrument, or the finger, and allow the pus to escape.

If the animal breathes with great difficulty, manifested by making a loud, wheezing sound, an opening should be made in his windpipe and the edges of the opening held apart by inserting a suture in each side, tying the silk ends up over the neck; or a tube may be inserted in the opening. This operation is called *tracheotomy.*

The sore-throat patient should never be drenched. If the horse should cough while taking medicine in this manner, the liquid might enter the lungs and cause pneumonia.

Fever may be combatted by cold-water injections into the rectum, 1 to 2 gallons at a time.

Strangles, Commonly Called "Distemper."

Strangles is an acute, infectious disease, and usually attacks young horses.

Symptoms. The disease begins with a high fever, ranging from 104° to 106°; a discharge from the nose, at first watery, rapidly becoming thicker, and later assuming a whitish-gray or greenish-yellow color. The glands below the lower jaw become swollen, hot, and painful, and occasionally there is soreness of the throat; loss of appetite, depression, great muscular weakness, and, occasionally, swelling of the hind legs follow. Sometimes a swelling may be found on some portion of the windpipe or other part of the body.

Treatment. Separate the sick animal from the healthy ones and place him in a well-ventilated stall, free from drafts; clean the nostrils frequently; clothe the body according to the season of the year; apply hot poultices to the abscess several times daily, and, as soon as pus is formed, open and wash twice daily.

Give easily digested food, green feed, roots, or slops made of bran or steamed oats, and to his drinking water add ½ ounce of saltpeter; do not drench, as the throat in many cases is sore.

Pneumonia.

Pneumonia is an inflammation of the lung structure, and usually runs a course of from seven to ten days.

Among the external causes of the disease are to be particularly mentioned excessive exertion and cold; also carelessness in giving a drench, particularly if the animal has a sore throat. This disease frequently follows acute nasal catarrh, sore throat or strangles, and may accompany influenza.

Symptoms. The first symptom is an intense fever accompanied by a chill; the patient shows great fatigue and muscular weakness; temperature ranges from 103° to 107°, the appetite is diminished, at times almost wanting; the patient is constipated; breathing is rapid and difficult; the nostrils are much dilated, and expired air is warmer than usual; the ears and legs are cold. There is frequently a rusty red or rusty yellow discharge from the nose. The animal remains standing constantly, with the fore legs spread, or it may lie down for a short time only; a cough may or may not be present.

Treatment. Great care should be given to the diet; in order to keep up his strength, give any food that the animal will eat — steamed oats, carrots, or green grass if possible, gruel, etc. Place him in a well-ventilated box stall free from drafts, and clothe the body and legs according to the season of the year; warm blankets wrapped around the chest if the weather is not too hot will be of advantage. In warm weather, if flies are troublesome, a thin sheet made of gunny sacks should be placed upon the animal. Quinine sulphate 1 dram, gentian root 2 drams, makes a good tonic. It should be repeated three times daily.

Cold injections into the rectum will reduce the fever.

Alcohol, 4 to 5 ounces, well diluted, should be given as a drench, twice daily, and potassium nitrate, ½ ounce, should be added to the drinking water.

In the first stage of pneumonia (called congestion of the lungs), caused by overexertion of the animal when he is in a weakened condition, the disease may be often broken up by the use of stimulants.

Heaves.

Heaves is a chronic disease of the lungs, manifested in a quick inspiration and a double expiration.

Symptoms. Cough of a chronic nature; discharge from the nostrils after exertion; characteristic breathing, as described above, which is aggravated by damp, muggy weather, and by dusty, coarse, and bulky fodder, such as clover hay or dirty oats. Climate has a marked influence; in high, dry altitudes this trouble is unknown.

Treatment. Always water before feeding, and feed more grain and less hay. The food must be clean, should be moistened before feeding, and the bowels should be kept loosened by frequent bran mashes. Never exercise a horse with heaves just after feeding.

Influenza (Pink Eye).

Influenza is a contagious disease. It affects first the respiratory tract, but also involves the nerve centers, circulatory system, the lining membranes of the intestines, and the eyes.

Symptoms. The first symptoms are loss of appetite, depression and weakness; the temperature rises rapidly to 105° or 107° in severe cases; the animal holds his head low and has a stupid look; he staggers when walking, and the visible mucous membranes are of a yellowish tinge.

When the digestive organs are affected, colics (gripes) occur frequently. In the beginning, constipation is the rule and the dung is coated with a whitish-yellow, mucus layer; later diarrhea occurs and the dung is doughy, soft, or liquid. The eyelids are sometimes swollen shut and are hot and sensitive to the touch. The legs and sheath are sometimes swollen and the lower portion of the belly may be similarly affected.

Treatment. Isolate sick animals for their own comfort and the safety of healthy subjects, as influenza is usually a serious disease. Give quinine sulphate 1 dram, gentian 2 drams, in a ball, three times daily; add ½ ounce saltpeter to the drinking water twice daily. The fever may be reduced by rectal injections of cold water.

Intestinal troubles may be relieved by the administration of bicarbonate of soda in dram doses three times daily; if pain is very severe, 2 drams of fluid extract of cannabis indica may be given. Bathe the eyes, if swollen, with warm water. Good nursing and laxative food are essential, cold water being kept where the animal can help himself.

CHAPTER VII

DISEASES OF THE DIGESTIVE, URINARY, NERVOUS, AND LYMPHATIC SYSTEMS

DISEASES OF THE DIGESTIVE SYSTEM

Spasmodic Colic – Gripes.

Spasmodic colic is a painful contraction of the intestines. The usual seat of the trouble is the small intestines, and it is usually caused by indigestible or chilled food or drink, and frequently by sudden chilling of the body.

Symptoms. The suffering is very violent but of short duration; the spasms appear suddenly and disappear with the same rapidity. The horse paws, stamps, looks around at his flanks, lies down and rolls, and if the pain is very severe, sweats profusely. During the attack a few pellets of dung may be passed, and attempts to pass urine are frequently made. This latter symptom has misled many persons to the impression that the disease was located in the "urinary organs."

Treatment. Place the animal in a large, well-bedded stall and give the following: Cannabis indica 2 to 4 drams, aromatic spirits ammonia 1 ounce, water to make 1 pint. Or, fluid extract belladonna 2 drams, nitrous ether 2 ounces, water to make 1 pint. Either one of these prescriptions can be given at one dose and repeated in three-quarters of an hour. If the animal is not relieved in one hour, give a purgative of aloes (physic ball).

Warm-water injections, per rectum, are often of advantage.

Flatulent Colic.

Flatulent colic is generally due to the animal having eaten improper foods, such as musty oats, sour bran, green corn, etc., which interfere with the process of digestion and give off much gas. It is sometimes caused merely by a sudden change of diet from oats to corn. This trouble is also frequently observed in horses that have the habit of wind sucking.

Symptoms. The rapid swelling of the belly constitutes the characteristic symptom. The abdomen is distended, the pain is not so severe as in spasmodic colic, but more constant. With the increase of swelling the breathing becomes more difficult, anxiety and restlessness are shown, walking is painful, and the animal staggers, lies down and rolls, but only for a short time.

Treatment. Place the horse in a large, roomy stall, and give the following drench: Sulphuric ether 2 ounces, aromatic spirits of ammonia 1 ounce, fluid extract belladonna 2 drams, water to make 1 pint. Repeat in one hour if necessary. Should the animal not be relieved after the second dose, administer a purgative. Cold-water injections into the rectum are sometimes of advantage. If the abdomen continues to distend with gas, the trocar and canula must be used. This is an instrument for puncturing the intestine, but should be used only by one who understands the operation. The instrument, as well as the seat of the operation, should be thoroughly disinfected.

51

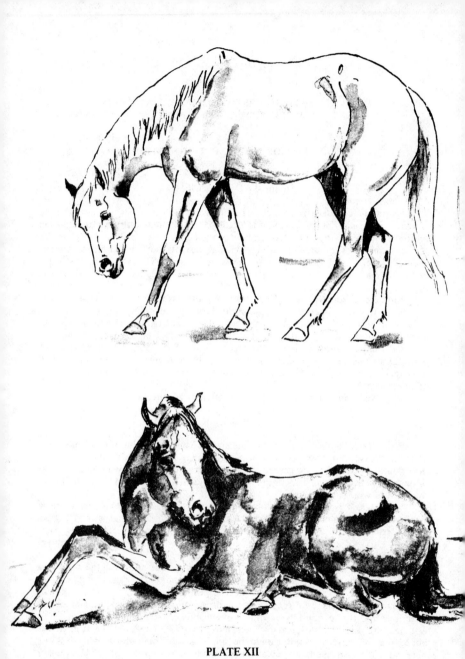

PLATE XII

Characteristic symptoms of spasmodic colic.

Enteritis — Inflammation of the Bowels.

Cause. This disease is sometimes due to the action of cold: sudden chilling when the body is in a perspiring condition, the swallowing of very cold water, of frozen or frost-covered fodder, etc. It is sometimes a complication of the colics and is frequently seen as a result of impaction or twisting of the bowels.

Symptoms. The mucous membrane of the nose, mouth, and eyes is congested and reddened, the mouth is hot and dry. Respiration is increased, pulse is hard and rapid, temperature is elevated, 103° to 105° F. Colicky pains are continuous; the horse walks about the stall, paws, lies down carefully, rolls, and *tries to balance himself on his back.* As a rule the bowels are constipated, but when this disease is due to irritating foods or medicines purgation and flatulency may be present.

The small, hard pulse; high temperature; aged and anxious appearance of the face; continuous pain, which is increased by pressure upon the abdomen; position of the horse when down, and coldness of the ears and legs, will enable anyone to diagnose a case of enteritis. When mortification (death) of the bowels sets in, all pain ceases and the animal will stand quietly, sometimes for several hours. Toward the last he sighs, breathes hard, staggers and pitches about, and dies in a state of delirium.

It is a very serious disease and in the majority of cases proves fatal. Death may take place in six hours, or not until after several days.

Treatment. To control the pain give large doses of powdered opium, laudanum, or cannabis indica.

The following prescription is recommended: Opium, powdered, 2 drams; calomel, ½ dram. Make into a ball; give at once, and repeat in one or two hours if necessary. Blankets wrung out in hot water and applied to the abdomen are sometimes of benefit, but to obtain good results they must be kept hot for several hours.

Chronic Indigestion.

Chronic indigestion is a chronic catarrh of the stomach and bowels, the causes of which are: Irregularity in feeding and watering; feeding when the animal is in an exhausted condition; imperfect mastication and incomplete salivation of food due to irregularities of the grinding surfaces of the molar teeth; and food of a poor quality, deficient in nutriment.

The presence of worms is a frequent cause of this disease.

Symptoms. Appetite diminished or capricious and depraved, frequent gaping, constipation; periodic colics are frequently observed, the coat is rough and staring, and the skin is tightly adherent to the body, the condition known as "hidebound." The animal has an unthrifty appearance generally.

Treatment. Give small quantities of good, nutritious, and well-salted food three times daily.

The water should be pure and given regularly.

Regular exercise and good grooming will hasten recovery, by stimulating the skin as well as other parts of the body.

If the appetite is diminished, give as a tonic: Gentian 2 ounces, iron sulphate 1 ounce, nux vomica 1½ ounces, nitrate potash 1½ ounces. Mix. Make twelve powders. Give one powder twice a day.

Bicarbonate of soda is a very useful medicine to counteract the acidity (sourness) of the stomach. Dose, 1 dram, twice a day; the doses may be continued for several days.

If intestinal worms are the exciting cause, they must be removed, and until this has been accomplished the animal will retain its unthrifty condition although it may brighten up temporarily.

The following prescription is recommended: Spirits turpentine 2 ounces, oil linseed 4 ounces. Give before feeding and repeat once a day for four days; then follow up with 1 pint of linseed oil.

Diarrhea.

This term is applied to all cases of simple purging in which the feces (dung) are loose, liquid, and frequently discharged.

Diarrhea may be a spontaneous effort to discharge from the intestines something which is obnoxious to them or to the system generally. It is caused by various agencies, such as indigestible food, sudden change of diet — particularly from a dry to a moist one — medicinal substances, worms, derangement of the liver, or large drafts of water when the animal is heated. Some animals are particularly predisposed to diarrhea from trivial causes. Narrow-loined, flat-sided, and loosely coupled horses — that is to say, horses in which the distance between the point of the hip and the last rib is long — and those of a nervous temperament are apt to purge without apparent cause. These are called *washy* horses. They are hard to keep in condition and require the best of food.

Symptoms. Purging, the fecal matter being semifluid, of a dirty-brown color, without offensive odor, or clay-colored and fetid. If the condition continues long the animal loses flesh and the appetite is wanting.

Treatment. When the purging arises from the presence of some offending matter in the intestinal canal (sand, worms, undigested food, etc.) its expulsion must be aided by a moderate dose of linseed oil (1½ pints).

If the purging arises from no apparent cause, or if the bowels do not regain their normal condition after the action of the oil has subsided, it will be necessary to give astringents (binding medicines), such as tannic acid, 1 to 2 drams. The following prescription may also be used: Gum camphor 1 ounce, opium, powdered, 1 ounce. Mix. Make eight powders and give one powder every three or four hours, according to the severity of the case. Great care must be exercised, as evil results may follow if the bowels are checked too soon.

DISEASES OF THE URINARY SYSTEM

Acute Nephritis — Inflammation of the Kidneys.

Causes. It is at times produced by the action of cold; it also happens frequently in the course of infectious (catching) diseases. The kidneys become irritated by the presence of waste materials of the food, such as mold, rust, etc., or by the passage of certain medicines, such as turpentine, cantharides, etc. Inflammation and partial or total clogging of the organ results. Cantharides will reach the kidneys after absorption from a large blistered surface.

Symptoms. The most important and often the only manifestations of nephritis (in the course of infectious diseases, for instance) are furnished by the urine. Its quantity is diminished; it is thickened; of abnormal color; occasionally it is the color of blood. Micturition (pissing) is painful; the urine often runs off drop by drop only, notwithstanding the violent efforts made by the patient. In serious cases the urinary secretion may be completely suppressed.

The lumbar region is very sensitive to the pressure of the hand. At the beginning of the disease we often have renal or kidney colics. The back is arched, the gait stiff and staggering, rising is painful; the animal remains almost constantly standing. The appetite may be lost. The temperature is elevated; in some cases it may range very high.

Treatment. Remove the cause if possible; avoid all irritating food or medicines, and give absolute rest. Try to induce sweating by energetic rubbings upon the surface of the whole body; also by warm blankets, and wet, tepid compresses applied upon the loins. Give the following physic: Aloes 6 drams, calomel 1 dram, ginger 1 dram. Make into a ball and give at one dose. It has a most favorable action, because the purging draws a large quantity of water from the system.

If there is a total suppression of urine, ½ ounce of fluid extract digitalis, well rubbed in on each side of the loins over the kidneys, will have a beneficial effect by stimulating the kidneys without causing irritation. This application should not be used more than once.

Diabetes Insipidus – Simple Diabetes (Pissing).

A disease characterized by great thirst, excessive urination, and great languor and emaciation.

In the majority of cases it is caused by poor and tainted food. In some cases it seems to be due to a constitutional cause.

Symptoms. Excessive urination, from 6 to 12 gallons every twenty-four hours; great thirst, the animal sometimes drinking from 20 to 25 gallons of water in twenty-four hours; depraved appetite; urine of a very pale color, sometimes as clear as water; the skin is harsh and the coat is unhealthy looking.

Treatment. Give good, clean, and nutritious food. Administer iodine in 1-dram doses three times a day and diminish quantity as the thirst is lessened and the urine is diminished.

Retention of the Urine.

An inability, total or partial, to expel by natural effort the urine contained in the bladder. It is caused by spasm of the neck of the bladder, and is often a complication of colic.

Symptoms. Frequent and ineffectual attempts to urinate; if standing the animal will stretch himself out, strain violently, and groan with pain, discharging but a few drops of urine, or none at all; by examination per rectum the bladder is felt to be greatly distended, and this is the diagnostic or distinguishing symptom.

Treatment. Pass the catheter and draw off the urine. If retention of the urine is due to an accumulation of dirt in the penis, washing will remove the cause.

DISEASES OF THE NERVOUS SYSTEM

Congestion of the Brain — "Blind Staggers."

This disease is caused by an accumulation of blood in the vessels of the brain, due to some obstacle to its return to the veins.

Causes. Disease of the heart; excessive exertion; the influence of extreme heat; sudden and great excitement; artificial stimulants; any mechanical obstruction which prevents the return of blood through the veins to the heart, such as a small ill-fitting collar; tumors or abscesses pressing on the vein in its course; extreme fat; compression of the vascular structures (arterial capillaries) by an abnormal tension of gas in the stomach and intestines; over-feeding after a prolonged abstinence or when the exercise is insufficient; and foods difficult of digestion. Fat horses or those with short, thick necks are especially liable to attacks of this malady.

Symptoms. Congestion of the brain usually appears suddenly and is of short duration.

The animal may stop very suddenly and shake his head, or stand quietly braced on his legs, then stagger, make a plunge and fall; the eyes are staring, breathing hurried and snoring, nostrils widely dilated; this may be followed by coma (insensibility), violent convulsive movement, and death.

Generally, however, the animal gains relief in a short time, but he may remain weak and giddy for several days. If it is due to organic change in the heart or disease of the blood vessels in the brain the symptoms may be of slow development, manifested by drowsiness, diminished or impaired vision, difficulty in voluntary movements, diminished sensibility of the skin, loss of consciousness, delirium, and death.

Treatment. Prompt removal of all mechanical obstruction to the circulation. If it is due to venous obstruction by too tight a collar, the loosening of the collar will give immediate relief. If due to tumors or abscesses, a surgical operation becomes necessary. To relieve the animal, if he becomes partially or totally unconscious, cold water should be dashed on the head, and if this does not afford relief, recourse must be had to bleeding to lessen arterial tension. If symptoms of paralysis remain after two or three days, an active physic should be given, followed, after twenty-four hours, by iodide of potassium given in 2-dram doses three times daily. Place the animal in a cool, dark well-ventilated stable, keep him perfectly quiet, and give cooling diet.

Sunstroke and Heatstroke.

These are cerebral troubles: Sunstroke is produced by the rays of the sun falling directly upon the cranium. Heatstroke is caused by the overheating of the whole body or by excessive exertion.

Symptoms. Sunstroke is manifested suddenly; the animal stops, drops his head, begins to stagger, the breathing is marked by great snoring, the pulse is very slow and irregular, cold sweats break out in patches on the surface of the body, and the animal often dies without recovering consciousness.

In heatstroke the animal usually requires urging for some time previous to the appearance of any other symptom. Generally perspiration is checked; he becomes weak in his gait; the breathing grows hurried or panting; the eyes watery and bloodshot; nostrils dilated and highly reddened to a dark purple color; the pulse is rapid and weak; the heart bounding, frequently followed by unconsciousness and death. Temperature reaches 107°F. to 112° F. If recovery takes place convalescence extends over a long period of time, during which locomotion shows lack of full control.

Treatment. The treatment consists in the application of cold in the form of ice or cold water on the head, cold injections per rectum, and the administration of stimulants, such as 2 ounces aromatic spirits of ammonia or 4 ounces of alcohol in 8 ounces of water; repeat in one hour if necessary. Place the animal in a cool and shady place, and bathe the whole body with cold water until the temperature is lowered.

DISEASES OF THE LYMPHATIC SYSTEM

Acute inflammation of the lymph gland usually occurs in connection with some inflammatory process in the region from which the lymph is gathered.

The lymph glands between the branches of the lower jaw almost invariably become affected in strangles, nasal catarrh (acute or chronic), diseased or ulcerated teeth. Infected wounds of any part of the body may cause inflammation of the neighboring lymphatics.

Symptoms. The glands swell and become painful to the touch, the connective tissue surrounding them becomes involved, suppuration (formation of pus) usually takes place, and one or more abscesses form. If the inflammation is of a milder type the swelling may disappear and the gland will assume its normal condition without suppuration. The temperature will be elevated. Sometimes the glands will remain hard and considerably swollen for some length of time. In man these swollen glands are known as kernels.

Treatment. Fomentations with hot water will relieve the soreness, unless an abscess is forming. If such is known to be the case a poultice of bran or flaxseed meal should be applied, and as soon as fluctuation can be felt a free opening must be made and the abscess washed with a solution of bichloride mercury 1-1000, or creolin 1-50. If the gland does not suppurate, the enlargement may be reduced by tincture of iodine applied twice daily.

Lymphangitis.

Inflammation of the lymphatic structures, usually affecting the hind leg, very seldom the fore leg. This disease is very sudden in its attack, exceedingly painful, accompanied by a high temperature and great general disturbance.

Causes. It usually attacks well-fed animals, especially after one or two days' rest, and in such cases may be due to an excess of nutritious elements in the blood. It may also result from an infected wound.

Symptoms. The first symptom noticed will be lameness in one leg and swelling on the inside of the thigh. The swelling gradually surrounds the whole limb, continuing downward until it reaches the foot. The limb is excessively tender to the touch and is held up. The breathing is increased, pulse hard and quick (80 to 100), and the temperature may reach 106°. The bowels early become constipated and the urine scanty and high colored. Occasionally the lymphatic glands in the groin undergo suppuration, blood poisoning may supervene and prove fatal.

Treatment. Fomentations with warm water, to be continued for one hour and repeated several times daily. Give a physic composed of 6 to 8 drams of aloes, 1 dram ginger, and water to make a ball. Give at once. After the physic has operated give ½-ounce doses of nitrate of potash twice daily. After the pain diminishes, moderate exercise and hand rubbing will be of benefit. If the glands suppurate, open, and wash them out with an antiseptic. The irrigations must be continued until the gland is well.

If caused by a wound, similar treatment should be pursued, together with thorough disinfection of the wound. If, after one week, the swelling still remains, give potassium iodide, 2 drams, twice daily until it is reduced.

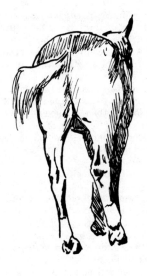

PLATE XIII

Lymphangitis.

CHAPTER VIII

MISCELLANEOUS DISEASES

PURPURA HEMORRHAGICA – PURPURA – PETECHIAL FEVER

This is an acute, infectious disease, the cause of which is as yet little known. Sometimes it is primary; in other instances it follows other infectious diseases, strangles, pharyngitis, contagious pneumonia, influenza, etc.

Symptoms. Petechial fever is generally manifested by the appearance upon the mucous membranes of numerous dark-red *petechiae* (reddish spots); sometimes they are insignificant as a flea bite, then again they may attain the size of a pea or an acorn; they often become joined and form spots or bands of variable length. In serious cases the nasal mucous membrane becomes affected by gangrene (death of the affected spot) or covered over with ulcerations. The discharge is bloody and of bad aspect, breathing is very laborious, and the expired air has a fetid odor. The general condition sometimes becomes very rapidly aggravated; then, in the majority of cases, the disease ends in death.

Corresponding with the appearance of the reddish spots, or a few days later, swellings appear beneath the skin; this symptom, which is the most prominent, is often the first symptom noticed. The swellings will range in size from a ten-cent piece to a silver dollar; they are usually upon dependent regions, such as the head, extremities, abdomen, sheath, and chest. These swellings are not hot, and only slightly sensitive; they gradually extend until they grow together, and we have in a few hours the swelling up of the legs and belly, or the head, to an enormous size; they have always a characteristic constricted border, which looks as if it had been tied with a cord. The swelling stands out abruptly at this border, often as much as an inch.

The swelling in the legs will cause stiffness. The head may be swollen to such a size that it resembles the head of a hippopotamus rather than that of a horse; the caliber of the nostril may be so lessened as to cause the horse to breathe with difficulty. The pulse, if altered at all, is a little weaker than usual, the appetite remains normal as a rule, although at times the animal will have difficulty in mastication. The temperature at first is normal, but in a few days it may have reached 102°, 103°, or 104°

Over the surface of the skin covering the swollen parts we find a slight serous sweating, which, when it dries, gives the appearance of an eruption of some cutaneous (skin) disease. If this is excessive we may see irritated spots, followed by suppuration. This suppuration may become excessive from the great distention and loss of vitality of the skin.

During the course of this disease colics may sometimes occur; later the pulse may beat 60 to 80 times per minute; the dung is ordinarily coated.

High temperatures indicate complications.

The mortality is about 50 per cent.

Treatment. Place the patient in a clean, well-ventilated, roomy box stall, and tie the head up *high*; in case the head is already swollen, remove the halter at once and use a head sling. If necessary to blanket never use the surcingle. Give soft food, clean hay, and green fodder, if possible, and plenty of fresh pure water to drink.

When the legs and parts of the body are covered by the dried serum the surface must be softened by the application of cosmoline or olive oil, to which may be added a small amount of creolin (1 to 50) or of carbolic acid (1 to 25).

If sloughing has taken place, the sores must receive surgical attention; dead tissue must be removed and antiseptics applied.

If the animal has great difficulty in breathing, we must resort to the use of the tracheotomy tube.

Try to sustain the strength of the animal and give tonics to increase the appetite: Tincture of chloride of iron 1 to 2 ounces in a pint of water, or iron sulphate 2 drams, quinine 1 dram; either dose three times daily.

Spirits of turpentine, 3 ounces, in 6 ounces of linseed oil, given twice daily, will have a beneficial effect by stimulating the heart and kidneys. Sponge the head, where swollen, with either ice-cold or very warm water; repeat this several times daily.

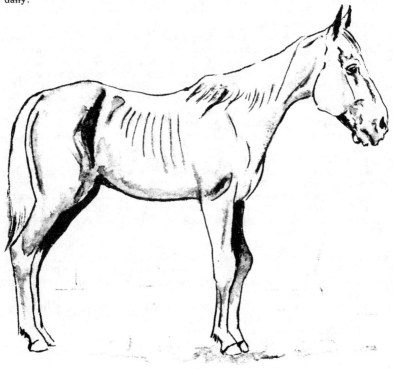

PLATE XIV

Purpura hemorrhagica.

AZOTURIA

Azoturia is the result of the confinement of a strong, vigorous horse for several days in a badly ventilated, damp stable, where he receives full rations and no exercise, followed by sudden exposure to a lower temperature. It is not a disease of the kidneys, as is commonly supposed.

Symptons. These consist of troubles of locomotion (movement), which appear during exercise and generally within a quarter to half an hour after starting.

The disease begins very suddenly, in an unusual degree of restlessness, with profuse perspiration; these symptoms are speedily succeeded by a desire to lie down, by great sluggishness, by loss of moving power in the hind limbs, and by violent spasms of the large muscle of the loins, thighs, and hind quarters. The affected muscles are swollen and very hard, and later may atrophy, especially those located above the stifle. If the animal is down, he makes an effort to stand, but, from the total loss of power in the hind limbs, is unable to rise.

The fore limbs and shoulder muscles may be similarly affected, but in this case the disease is less severe.

The pulse usually becomes rapid; the temperature rarely increases, even in the grave form; the appetite is seldom diminished, and, as a rule, the animal will drink large quantities of water.

The urine is *coffee-colored* and is generally retained in the bladder.

Treatment. As soon as the first symptoms are noticed, *halt at once.* Keep the animal on his feet; unsaddle or unharness and blanket promptly; then move him as gently as possible to the nearest shelter, where he must have complete rest. If possible, heat some common salt or some oats; place in a sack and spread over the loins (under the blanket), to relieve the pain. Feed only good hay or laxative food and avoid oats and corn. Encourage the horse to drink as much water as possible, as this will assist the kidneys in carrying the poisonous material out of the blood. When the urine clears, the animal may be gradually returned to work.

If it has been possible to reach the stables, place the horse in a roomy stall; if there is then danger of his lying down, use the suspending slings, provided he is able to partially support his weight on his hind legs; then give 2 ounces of sweet spirits of niter and 2 to 4 drams of fluid extract of cannabis indica in a pint of water. In a half hour administer a physic ball.

If the animal has dropped on the road and is unable to rise he must be taken to the stable by the use of a stone boat or other extemporized means; plenty of bedding must then be supplied and the patient frequently turned from side to side; apply ½ ounce of fluid extract of digitalis to the loins and rub in well, to simulate the action of the kidneys. If the patient has retention of urine, the bladder must be emptied several times daily; this can be accomplished by passing the hand into the rectum and applying moderate pressure upon the bladder, or by the introduction of the catheter.

This disease occurs only through carelessness. When the horse is left resting for twenty-four to forty-eight hours or longer the food ration should be diminished, and the animal must be given a little exercise in the open air every day to keep him accustomed to the outside temperature.

GLANDERS AND FARCY

Glanders is a contagious constitutional disease of the horse and mule, and may be communicated to man. The disease is due to a germ called "bacillus mallei," and affects the Schneiderian membrane and internal organs.

When the disease is located in the lymphatic glands situated on the external parts of the body it is called farcy.

Glanders and farcy are one and the same disease.

It may be acute or chronic. In acute glanders the bacilli enter the blood and the disease spreads throughout the system.

Chronic glanders.

The beginning of chronic glanders is often hidden from view and passes unobserved.

The first visible symptom is generally a discharge from one or both nostrils of a yellowish green matter of bad aspect; quite frequently it is tinged with blood.

Then pimples and ulcers are observed upon the Schneiderian membrane. The pimples are of short duration; they are soon transformed into ulcers more or less deep, with sawtooth-shaped, thickened edges; these may heal, but will always leave a scar.

The enlargement of the lymphatic glands situated in the space between the lower jaw is another important symptom. In the beginning the gland is a little sensitive, slightly doughy, and adheres to the base of the tongue or to the lower maxillae; in some subjects it adheres to the skin. In exceptional cases the enlargement of the gland is absent.

The general health of the animal suffers as the affection progresses; emaciation appears; the hair becomes dull and bristly.

There is frequently difficulty in breathing, and the patient becomes rapidly fatigued.

Farcy.

Farcy is more rare in the chronic than in the acute form of the disease; its favorite regions are the inner side of the extremities, shoulders, neck, chest, and abdomen.

The pimples and tumors vary from the size of a pea to that of a walnut, or larger; they suppurate and discharge a yellow, sticky liquid of bad aspect. They rarely heal, and if they do a jagged scar remains.

Symptoms. Acute glanders is rare in the *horse* (10 per cent), except in transit and in tropical climates. It is, on the contrary, the ordinary form in the mule. Sometimes it is primary; in other instances it follows the chronic form, where the vitality of the animal has been lessened by other acute affections.

The disease produces an ulcerous destruction of the respiratory mucous membrane, and also involves the skin, lungs, and other organs.

It begins with a chill, followed by intense fever, which reaches 107° F. A. sticky, yellowish, irritating, bloody nasal discharge appears. The nasal mucous membrane is overrun with pimples and ulcers, which rapidly join one another; they may perforate the septum nasi. The respiration is rattling, wheezing, and moaning, due to contraction of the larynx; to these symptoms are often added those of farcy. We may find diarrhea. The patient is extremely weak and emaciation progresses rapidly.

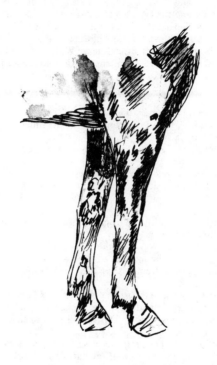

PLATE XV
Farcy

63

In general, acute glanders runs a rapid course; its usual termination is death. This ordinarily takes place within from three to fourteen days.

In the horse there is no disease of which an exact diagnosis is so important as that of glanders.

In order to correctly diagnose obscure cases (those with no outward symptoms), we must resort to the use of mallein. This is a liquid, the injection of which will cause a reaction (rise in temperature) in glandered horses apparently enjoying the best of health.

Treatment. This disease is not only contagious to horses, mules, and men, but is *incurable* in all alike; therefore, the first step, when a suspicious case presents itself, is to isolate the animal, and as soon as it is proved that glanders exists, the animal should be killed at once and the carcass burned. Everything in the way of partitions, mangers, feed boxes, buckets, and all stable utensils must be burned, and the stalls and surroundings thoroughly disinfected. Chloride of lime, 8 ounces in 1 gallon of water, makes a good and efficient disinfectant. With this solution all parts of the stable in which the affected animal stood must be thoroughly washed.

TETANUS—LOCKJAW

Tetanus is an infectious disease, the specific cause of which is a bacillus or germ which, in most localities, is found in abundance in the superficial layer of the earth in gardens, around buildings, stables, etc.

The disease, when present, always follows a wound, more especially one produced by a nail puncture.

The germ will not develop in the presence of oxygen; consequently, all punctured wounds of the foot should be freely opened to admit of the introduction of air, as well as to allow of thorough cleansing with an antiseptic. This preventive treatment is generally successful.

In warm countries, especially in tropical climates, cases of tetanus are much more frequent than in cold regions.

Symptoms. Tetanic spasms (spasmodic or continuous contractions of the muscles) appear, as a rule, in the muscles of the neck and head; thence they extend to the shoulders, trunk, and extremities; or the stiffness may start in the region of the injured organ or member.

Contraction of the cheek muscles; the inferior maxillary is then no longer able to execute the slightest movement, and the prehension and mastication of food becomes difficult or quite impossible. This inability to open the jaws has given to the disease the name of lockjaw.

Contraction of the great posterior muscles of the eye causes a retraction of this organ within the orbit, and a protrusion of the haw upon the eyeball.

The animal is very stiff, holds his head in an extended position as if suffering from a sore throat; the tail is elevated and the ears drawn closer together; the nostrils are much dilated; the legs stand apart; the eyes indicate excitement and anxiety, the mucous membranes are reddened; some muscular groups, principally the muscles of the cheeks and of the back of the neck, are hard and distinctly outlined, as if carved; the muscles of the jaws, neck and shoulders, back, lumbar region, croup and tail are as hard as wood.

The tail and ears may be moved by the hand, but they immediately return to their former position.

There is profuse sweating when the animal is disturbed, or when he is in a spasm; respiration is accelerated and laborious. When the patient is approached for

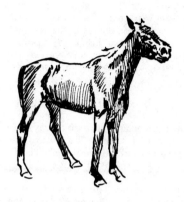

PLATE XVI

Tetanus.

an examination, his excitement increases instantly. The lower jaw is pressed hard against the upper, and can not be separated from it, even by the most violent efforts of the examiner; on parting the lips a fetid liquid runs out of the mouth, which is more or less filled with particles of food; if the head is lifted the whole haw obscures the greater part of the eyeball.

Backing is extremely difficult or even impossible; turning is also very laborious; the trunk, neck, and shoulders can not be flexed, the extremities are as stiff as stilts.

The course of tetanus is variable, according to the individual. It commonly develops rapidly, and death takes place in two or three days. In some cases death occurs more slowly, within four to eight days on an average. In others, again, where the spasm is moderate and of little extent, the disease may continue for several weeks.

Recovery before the third week is rare; about this time the spasm begins to decline, the appetite returns, respiration becomes calmer, and the movements more free; very often recovery takes place only at the end of five or six weeks; there may be a continuance of the stiffness of movement and tension of the muscles of the back for a long period of time.

Treatment. A systematic course of food and the freedom of the patient from all kinds of excitement are the two essentials in the treatment.

It is advisable to place the patient in a dark stall, so situated as to be isolated and free from all noises, and with only one man in attendance; strangers entering the stall of a patient affected with only a mild attack may cause such excitement that the animal is thrown into a violent spasm and dies in a short time.

Give the patient gruel, mealy drinks, liquid food, and, if he can eat it, green fodder.

Medicinal agents are of secondary importance in the treatment of lockjaw. Large doses (2 to 8 ounces) of bromide of potassium should be given in the liquid food, twice daily. The administration of medicines by the mouth is not practicable; not only because of the locked jaws, but because it causes excitement.

The infected wound requires special care. It should be well opened up, disinfected, foreign bodies extracted, etc.

Some authorities recommend the use of the suspending sling.

In the horse the mortality from this disease is from 80 to 85 per cent.

In localities where tetanus is common, a preventive serum, called "antitetanic," is injected into the blood, whenever the horse receives a punctured or suspicious wound.

DISEASES OF THE TEETH

On account of the character of its food the horse has been supplied with molar teeth, with roughened grinding surfaces. The lower jaw is narrower than the upper jaw, and the table (grinding) surfaces are sloping. The distance from the gum to the grinding surface is greater on the outside surface of the upper molars and the reverse in the lower molars.

On account of this conformation a sharp ridge of points is liable to develop on the outside of the upper molars and may occur on the inside of the lower ones. These points are sometimes so sharp that they lacerate the cheeks and tongue during mastication. A horse thus affected will frequently bolt his food before thoroughly masticating it, thereby causing chronic indigestion. He will also flinch when reined, causing great annoyance to his rider or driver.

Such irregularities can be easily detected by an examination of the animal's mouth with the hand; when found, the sharp edges must be removed by the use of a float.

Decayed teeth.

All teeth are apt to decay, such decay being generally due to an injury.

A decayed tooth will be found in one of the following conditions: Split, broken, or shorter than the surrounding ones, and having a fetid odor. The opposing tooth in the opposite jaw is often found to be elongated.

Symptoms of irregularities in teeth. Quidding of the food, holding the head to one side while masticating food or drinking water, slobbering, chronic catarrh, fetid breath, swelling of the maxilla in the neighborhood of the teeth, general unthrifty appearance, etc.

Treatment. A diseased tooth must be extracted, and an elongated one must be shortened to correspond with its fellows.

SPASM OF THE DIAPHRAGM – THUMPS

Caused by severe exertion.

Symptoms. In the region of the lower part of the left flank, near the border of the false ribs, will be observed shocks which, at times, shake the whole body; they are usually accompanied by a short, jerking expiration, and by a dull, thumping sound which is heard at a distance of several paces. The trouble may be followed by inflammation of the lungs or by founder.

Treatment. Absolute quiet and fresh air free from draughts.

Give the following: Aromatic spirits ammonia 2 ounces, water 1 pint. Or, sweet spirits of niter 2 ounces, fld. ext. belladonna 2 drams, water to make 1 pint. Either mixture may be repeated in one hour if necessary.

If inflammation of the lungs or founder follows, treat accordingly.

CHAPTER IX

DISEASES OF THE SKIN AND EYE

ERYTHEMA

Erythema is a slightly inflamed condition of the skin, unattended by any eruption. The parts are slightly swollen, hot, tender, or itchy, and dry, and if the skin is white there is redness.

Erythema may arise from a variety of causes, as chilling or partial freezing, heat and burning, chapping, urine, and medicine.

Treatment. Apply the following several times daily: Sulphate of zinc 1 ounce, acetate of lead 1 ounce, water 1 quart. Or, use the following ointment twice daily: Oxide of zinc 1 ounce, cosmoline 6 ounces.

GREASE

Grease is a chronic inflammation of the skin of the back part of the fetlock and pastern. It is usually caused by lack of cleanliness, but may result from overfeeding without exercise.

The skin is at first red, swollen, painful, and hot. It is soon covered by vesicles (blisters) which burst and discharge a thin, yellowish liquid, which is at first without odor. The hairs are matted together, erect, or fall out in large quantities.

Grease produces, in the course of time, serious alterations in the pastern or fetlock. The excreted liquid becomes decomposed and softens the epidermis. A kind of sticky, doughy exudate is formed, which is of bad aspect, of fetid odor, and very irritating.

The back part of the pastern and fetlock becomes the seat of granulating wounds, the granulations ranging in size from that of a pea to a large grape (the so-called grapy stage).

Treatment. In the first stage cleanliness and the application of the ordinary drying powder or antiseptic ointments are sufficient. In cases where proud flesh exists, the granulations must be removed with the knife and burned with red-hot iron or lunar caustic and then treated as a fresh wound. Applications of iodine and glycerin in equal parts, or of the three sulphates, may be beneficial.

SCRATCHES

Scratches is allied to grease and results from similar causes; it is not so severe, but if neglected may terminate in that disease. It is usually of a dry nature, with shallow cracks in the skin, and often discharging a thin liquid, which does not irritate the skin. The disease is located in the back part of the pastern joint.

Treatment. Cleanse thoroughly with castile soap and water, dry, and apply: Sulphate of zinc 1 ounce, acetate of lead 1 ounce, water 1 quart. Or, oxide of zinc 1 part, lanolin 10 parts. Or, tincture of iodine may be resorted to. Good results are obtained by a dressing of equal parts of zinc oxide and acetanilid, kept in place by a piece of gauze or cotton and a bandage.

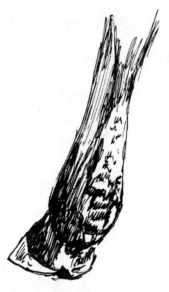

PLATE XVII

Grease.

SCABIES – MANGE

This is a contagious skin disease produced by parasites and can be transmitted to man.

There are three parasites that cause mange; two varieties burrow into the deeper layers of the skin, the first being found about the head and neck (though it may spread over the surface of the body), the second at the roots of the mane and tail; the third species does not burrow into the skin and is found on the extremities.

Symptoms. This disease is characterized by great itching associated with the formation of pustules (pimples). As the disease develops, large surfaces become destitute of hair and are covered by powdery crusts of variable thickness. At a later period the skin becomes thickened, wrinkled, and fissured, assuming the appearance of the skin of the rhinoceros.

Treatment. The first essential is the separation and isolation of the unhealthy from the well animals. Wash the affected parts thoroughly with warm water, soap, and a scrubbing brush, and apply the following: Acetanilid 10 parts, creolin 5 parts, cosmoline 20 parts. Melt the cosmoline and mix with the other ingredients while cooling. This ointment should be applied twice a day and the parts thoroughly washed every other day. Continue the treatment until the skin becomes healthy.

SIMPLE INJURIES TO THE EYELIDS

Inflammation of the mucous membrane lining the eyelids may be caused by bruises or the presence of a foreign body, such as sand, chaff, etc. If the eyelids should become torn, they must be sutured; the utmost care is necessary as the needle may puncture the eyeball and blindness will follow.

Treatment. Keep the parts clean with a saturated solution of boracic acid, and dust with iodoform.

SIMPLE OPHTHALMIA – CONJUNCTIVITIS

Inflammation of the outer parts of the eyeball, and of the exposed vascular, sensitive mucous membrane (conjunctiva) which covers the ball, the eyelids, and the haw.

The causes of external ophthalmia are mainly those which act locally – blows with whips, clubs, and twigs; the presence of foreign bodies, such as chaff, dust, sand, ammonia arising from the excrement, etc.

Symptoms. Watering of the eye, swollen lids, redness of the mucous membrane exposed by the separation of the lids, and a bluish opacity of the cornea, which normally is clear and transparent. The eyelids may be kept closed, the eyeball retracted, and the haw protruded over one-third or one-half of the ball. If the affection has resulted from a wound of the cornea, a white speck or fleecy cloud is formed, and often blood vessels begin to extend from the adjacent vascular covering of the eye to the white spot, and that portion of the cornea is rendered permanently opaque.

Treatment. Place the horse in a dark stall and bathe the outside of the eye with tepid water; a few drops of the following lotion should be dropped inside the eyelids: Zinc sulphate 20 grains, boracic acid 1 dram, fluid extract of belladonna 1 dram, water 4 ounces. Cover the eye with a clean, dark cloth on the inside of which a piece of absorbent cotton has been sewed; keep the cotton saturated with the same lotion. This treatment should be applied and continued twice daily until the parts assume their normal condition. In case of wound or ulcer on the cornea, make use of a quill, through which blow iodoform into the eye daily.

RECURRENT OPHTHALMIA – MOONBLINDNESS

This affection, sometimes called periodic ophthalmia, is an inflammation of the interior of the eye; it is intimately related to certain soils and climates, and to certain animal systems, in which it shows a strong tendency to recur again and again, usually ending in blindness from cataract or other serious injury. Continuous exposure to bright sunlight is frequently an exciting cause.

Symptoms vary according to the severity of the attack. In some cases there is marked fever. The local symptoms are in the main those of simple ophthalmia; opacity advances from the margin over a part or the whole of the cornea. An attack lasts from ten to fifteen days. The attacks may follow each other at intervals of a month, more or less, but they show no particular relation to any particular phase of the moon. From five to seven attacks usually result in blindness, and then the other eye is liable to be attacked until it also is ruined.

71

Treatment. Is largely the same as that for simple ophthalmia. During recovery a course of tonics is often very beneficial and acts in assisting to ward off another attack. Such a tonic is the following: Sulphate iron 1 ounce, gentian 1½ ounces, nux vomica 1½ ounces. Make into twelve powders and give one powder, in feed, twice a day.

If opacity of the cornea remains, benefit may be obtained from the use of silver nitrate, 4 grains to 1 ounce of water, a few drops dropped into the eye twice daily. A saturated solution of iodide of potassium may be used in the same manner.

CATARACT

Cataract is usually the result of repeated attacks of recurrent ophthalmia. It is an opacity, not of the cornea, but of the *crystalline lens.* No treatment will restore it to its normal condition.

CHAPTER X

DISEASES OF THE FEET

Removing pressure means trimming the bearing surfaces of the foot in such a way that the shoe can not cause pressure upon diseased structures.

CORNS

A corn is the result of bruising the sensitive sole or sensitive laminae of the quarters or bars and appears as a reddish spot in the angle formed by the wall and bar, usually on the inside of the front feet, seldom, if ever, in the hind feet.

Causes. A rapid gait on hard roads; lowering one quarter more than the other; shoes so fitted that they press on the sole at the heel, and shoes left on so long that the wall overgrows the heels of the shoe and causes the shoe to press on the sole; long feet, which remove the frog too far from the ground, thus preventing the proper expansion of the foot.

Treatment. First remove the cause by taking off the shoe; shorten the toe, lower the quarter that is too high, or correct any faults that may have existed in the preparation of the foot. Remove all pressure from the affected spot and reshoe.

In case of severe inflammation and probable suppuration, poultice or soak the foot until the horn softens and pus appears; open freely, disinfect, remove all horn that is underrun by pus and then pack with the "three sulphates" until suppuration ceases. Plug the corn with oakum or tar and shoe with a bar shoe, removing all pressure from the affected quarter. (The special function of the bar shoe is to produce frog pressure.) The three-quarter shoe may also be used. This shoe will prevent pressure on the diseased spot, but it has a tendency to give a rocking motion to the foot in action.

THRUSH

Thrush is a diseased condition of the frog, characterized by a dark-colored discharge of offensive odor.

Causes. Uncleanliness; horses standing in stalls saturated with urine, or in wet earth filled with decomposing vegetable matter.

Symptoms. At first there is simply an increased moisture in the cleft of the frog, accompanied by an offensive smell. After a time the discharge is more profuse, then watery and highly offensive, changing gradually to a thick, putrid matter, which rapidly destroys the horn of the frog.

Treatment. Remove the cause; keep stalls clean and dry. Pare away all loose portions of the horn, so as to expose the diseased parts; clean thoroughly by washing with warm water; dry with oakum and pack with powdered alum, calomel, or copper sulphate; if the dressing will not remain in place use a leather boot.

CANKER

Canker is a disease of the frog and sole, marked by an offensive-smelling, cheesy discharge, by a softening and breaking down of the horny frog and sole, and a spongy enlargement of the sensitive frog and sole. When this disease follows an injury which has exposed the soft structures of the foot, it soon causes a separation of the soft and horny portions, presenting a very unhealthy appearance and discharging a thin, watery fluid.

Causes. Canker is generally believed to be caused by a vegetable parasite, the development of which is assisted by filthy stables or low, wet ground.

Treatment. That part of the frog or sole that has been underrun must be removed with the knife and the canker exposed; the unhealthy growth is then touched with a red-hot iron, burning it off level with the surrounding healthy structures, care being exercised not to injure the sensitive portions of the foot. Next, wash clean, then dry and apply the following powder: Equal parts of sulphate of zinc, sulphate of iron, and sulphate of copper. Place over this a pad of oakum, and over all a leather boot. This dressing must be changed once a day (twice a day in bad cases); treatment is continued until a healthy growth of horn covers the whole foot. The horse can now be shod. Pack the foot with oakum and tar and cover with a leather sole, which is held in place by the shoe.

If it is desirable to change dressings on the shod foot, a more convenient appliance to keep them in place is made in the following manner: Cut a piece of sheet zinc to cover about two-thirds of the sole and frog, the outer edge of the piece fitting under the shoe; cut another piece to cover the remaining third and wide enough to lap over the first piece, the lap to run parallel to the cleft of the frog; then cut a strip about 1 inch wide to act as a keeper; the ends of this strip are pressed under the shoe, the strip passing across the foot from quarter to quarter.

QUITTOR

A quittor is a running sore, situated on the coronet of the foot, with one or more tubes (sinuses) leading in a downward direction and discharging pus.

Causes. Pricks in shoeing: punctures of the coronet, sole or frog; bruises or suppurating corns.

Symptoms. A swelling on the coronet, presenting a peculiarly unhealthy appearance, and in the center of which are one or more sinuses communicating with the diseased structures inside of the foot. In nearly all cases the horse is very lame.

Treatment. Find out, if possible, what has caused the quittor. If it is the result of a nail prick or a festered corn, open it up on the underside of the foot, allow the pus to run out, and then treat as described under "Puncture." If no nail prick or corn can be found, treat the quittor from above, by injecting into the sinuses one of the following solutions: Carbolic acid, 1 to 20; creolin, 1 to 25; bichloride of mercury, 1 to 500. This treatment should be continued for several days, at the end of which period, if the parts do not appear in a healthier condition, inject into the tubes 1 dram of bichloride of mercury well shaken up in 1 ounce of water. This will cause a separation of the diseased walls of the tube from the healthy parts of the foot. Poultices of flaxseed meal assist this separation. Keep the parts clean and wash out with carbolic acid or creolin as at first. If the sore does not heal under this treatment a surgical operation will be necessary.

QUARTER CRACKS AND TOE CRACKS

A toe or quarter crack (often called a sand crack) is a split in the horn of the wall; the position of the crack determines the name applied to it. Horses with thin, weak quarters are predisposed to quarter crack.

Causes. Excessive dryness of the hoof; alternate changing from damp to dry; heavy shoes; large nails, and nails set too far back toward the heels.

Symptoms. The crack generally starts at the coronary band and gradually extends downward to the lower border of the wall. The most common form of quarter crack is a deep fissure extending through the wall and causing a pinching of the sensitive structures. When, however, the crack is not deep there is seldom any lameness.

Treatment. The first step is to remove the shoe and soften the horn by poultices or by standing in warm or cold water for a few days, then cut away the hard overlapping edges of the fissure and thin the wall on each side so that there will be no friction between the edges of the crack. As the wall grows down from the coronet the upper end of the crack must be carefully observed to see that the new horn grows down strong and smooth. In time the crack will disappear at the lower edge of the wall. If the sensitive laminae have been exposed by this operation, the parts should be washed with a solution of creolin, 1 to 50, and the wound should be dusted with acetanilid and covered with a pad of oakum held in place by a boot or bandage. In a few days a thin layer of horn will be thrown out, covering the sensitive laminae. The horse can then generally be put to work.

After a quarter crack has been trimmed out, the horse should be shod with a bar shoe, the wall underneath the quarter crack being cut away so that it will not come in contact with the shoe.

In a case of toe crack the operation is the same. In shoeing, the wall is cut away at the toe to prevent pressure.

PUNCTURE OF THE SOLE AND FROG – PRICKS IN SHOEING

A puncture of the sole or frog is usually caused by a horse stepping on a nail, a piece of broken glass, or other sharp object. If the wound enters the soft structures of the foot, it results in lameness and the formation of pus.

Pricks in shoeing are of two kinds: First, when the nail is driven into the soft structures, and, second, when it is driven too close, causing a bulging of the inner layer of horn, which is forced in upon the sensitive laminae. In the first case the horse goes lame immediately; in the second case lameness may not appear for several days or weeks.

To detect a punctured wound of the foot remove the shoe, examining each nail as it is withdrawn for traces of moisture. Then test with the pinchers. When the sore spot is pressed, the horse will flinch.

Treatment. Open the wound and let out any pus that may have formed; wash out with a solution of creolin, 1 to 25, or of carbolic acid, 1 to 20. Unless the pus has a good outlet, it will burrow into the surrounding tissues and quittor or canker may follow. Moreover, there is always danger of tetanus in all cases of punctured wounds, especially in the feet. The germ of this disease is present in nearly all soils and is very liable to be carried into the wound upon the nail or other object. After the wound has been opened up and washed out, the foot should be placed in a hot flaxseed poultice, a fresh one being applied three or four times a day, and the parts washed out after each poultice, as in the first instance. The treatment should be continued until inflammation is reduced and the formation of pus has ceased. The hole can then be plugged with oakum and tar, the shoe reset, and the horse put to work.

LAMINITIS OR FOUNDER

Laminitis is an inflammation of the sensitive laminae (generally of the front feet) and may involve the adjoining structures. There are three forms of the disease — acute, subacute, and chronic.

The exudation of blood is greatest at the toe, the foot being more vascular at that point. The pain of acute laminitis is very persistent and agonizing, because the swollen and sensitive portions of the foot are surrounded by the hard and unyielding hoof and the engorged blood vessels are not permitted free exudation and swelling, the normal means by which congested blood vessels are relieved.

Causes. The most common are concussion, overexertion, exhaustion, rapid changes of temperature, the eating of various improper foods, such as musty grain, hay, etc., and the drinking of cold water when the animal is overheated.

Symptoms. In acute laminitis of both front feet the animal is excessively lame, moves with great difficulty, especially when starting, and appears as if the entire body were in a state of cramp; he stands with the hind legs drawn under the belly and the fore feet advanced, in order to relieve them of as much weight as possible. Occasionally he may be seen to sway backward, elevating the toes and throwing the weight for a moment upon the heels of the front feet, and then resuming the original position. If compelled to move, he raises the feet laboriously, not because the muscles of locomotion are inflamed, as is sometimes supposed, but because, if all four feet are not on the ground at the same time to bear the weight of the body, his suffering is increased. He will often groan with pain and sweat will break out over the body. To diagnose a case quickly, the best method is to push the horse backward, when, if affected, he will elevate the toes and throw his weight upon the heels.

The pulse in acute laminitis is full, strong, and rapid and will maintain these characteristics even after general debility has become manifest. In some instances the animal will lie down upon his side, with legs stretched out, for hours at a time, evidently feeling great relief in this position; in other cases, particularly during the early period of the disease, he will stand persistently. The temperature ranges from 102° to 104°.

Treatment. Remove the shoes from the affected feet; stand the horse in hot water for several hours each day, or, what is equally good and perhaps safer, apply hot flaxseed poultices, changing them every hour as they become cold. After two or three days of this treatment change to cold water, which can be applied either in the form of a footbath or by standing the animal in a running stream for five or six hours at a time. As soon as the pain has diminished, moderate exercise is beneficial; this may be gradually increased until the animal shows no further sign of trouble. If, after five or six days, pronounced symptoms of recovery are not apparent, apply a stiff blister of cantharides around the coronet, repeating the blister if necessary. In addition to the local treatment, nitrate of potash (saltpeter), in doses of 2 to 4 ounces, may be given three times a day. If the horse is constipated, give 1 quart or raw linseed oil. The subacute and chronic forms may be relieved by softening the foot as in "Dry feet," by occasional blistering and by intelligent shoeing.

SEEDY TOE

Seedy toe is a mealy condition of the inner wall of the hoof, the white line, and sometimes the sole. It is most frequently seen in the front feet.

Causes. Undue pressure, clips on shoes, or the result of laminitis.

Treatment. Pare the wall of the cavity until healthy horn is reached and pack with tar and oakum. Stimulate healthy growth of horn by the application of a cantharides blister at the coronet. Omit the clip in reshoeing.

CONTRACTED FEET

Contracted feet is an unnatural shrinking or narrowing of the feet at the heels. Most often seen in the front feet.

Causes. Lack of exercise; lack of moisture; thrush; shoes with bearing web inclining inward at the heels. The practice of using the knife to "open the heels" usually produces this trouble.

Treatment. Ascertain the cause and remove it if possible. The remedy is to secure normal pressure on the frog, bars, and heels. If the feet are extremely dry and hard they may be softened by standing the animal in moist clay or in water. If the character of the ground will permit let the horse go barefoot; if not, shoe with the tip, preferably; otherwise, with the bar shoe.

DRY FEET

Soften the hoofs by thorough soaking in water *and then* apply cosmoline or linseed oil to prevent the water from evaporating. This should be done daily for a week or two. A thick paste of ground flaxseed and water, packed into the cavity of the foot between the branches of the shoe, or a packing of moist clay, will keep the foot soft.

COFFIN-JOINT LAMENESS

Sprain of the coffin joint results from slipping, stepping upon a rolling stone, stepping into a hole, etc.

Symptoms. Shortened gait; lameness and pointing of diseased foot; heat over the region of the coffin joint; tenderness on pressure.

Treatment. Remove the shoe and give the animal complete rest; poultice the foot with flaxseed meal or stand the foot in a tub of cold water; if relief is not obtained in a week, apply a blister of biniodide of mercury, 1 to 5, around the coronet and heels, rubbing it in well over the region of the heels.

Sprain of the coffin joint, unless carefully nursed, may terminate in chronic *navicular disease,* in which the coffin-joint structures and the coffin bone itself become ulcerated. This disease is incurable.

If, after navicular disease has developed, it is necessary to keep the horse in the service, the heel of the diseased foot should be elevated by the use of a shoe with calks or with thick heels. The foot should be kept soft with footbaths and poultices and a blister applied when lameness is especially marked. Whenever possible keep the shoe off during treatment.

CHAPTER XI

DISEASES OF BONE AND DETECTION OF LAMENESS

SIDEBONES

Sidebones is an ossification (turning into bone) of the lateral cartilage. Horses with flat feet and weak quarters are predisposed to this disease.

Symptoms. A hard, unyielding condition of the lateral cartilage, with or without lameness.

Treatment. If the horse is lame the first step is to remove the shoe and level the foot; then let the horse stand in a tub of cold water for several hours a day, or apply, around the coronet, swabs kept wet with cold water. As soon as the fever has disappeared clip off the hair over the sidebones and blister with this ointment: Biniodide of mercury 1 part, cosmoline 5 parts; mix thoroughly and rub in for ten minutes. Tie up the horse's head so that he can not reach the blistered part with his lips, and keep him in this position for twenty-four to forty-eight hours. Then wash off the blister, using warm water and castile soap. The washing must be repeated every day until all the scabs formed by the blister have been removed. During this time keep the horse standing quietly in a clean and level stall. If after ten days he has not improved, firing, followed by a long period of rest, may prove beneficial.

RINGBONE

Ringbone is a bony enlargement, more or less prominent, situated upon either the os suffraginis or os coronae, and it may also involve the articular cartilages.

Causes. Blows, sprains, jumping, fast work on hard roads, and faulty conformation.

Symptoms. Lameness is usually the first symptom, and diagnosis is assisted by palpation (feeling) and comparison of the two legs. The enlargement is hard, painless on pressure, and the skin covering is movable.

Treatment. The foot must be pared perfectly level and a blister applied to the enlargement and repeated in two weeks if necessary. Perfect rest and quietude for four to six weeks are essential, or no beneficial results can be expected.

If the rest and blisters fail to remove the lameness firing may sometimes be resorted to. Puncture firing in two or three rows is often very effective. After firing the seat of the injury should be blistered with biniodide of mercury, 1 to 5, and the animal kept quiet in a single stall for at least one month.

BONE SPAVIN

Bone spavin is a disease involving the bones in the hock joint and is usually manifested in a bony enlargement, situated at the inner and lower part of the tarsus.

Causes. Weakness, faulty conformation, severe strains, hard and rapid work, etc.

Symptoms. The appearance of this disease is usually accompanied by lameness, which in the early stages of the disease is noticed only when the animal is first moved after a rest, and then the toe is generally placed upon the ground first. When standing, the animal often rests the diseased leg on the toe.

79

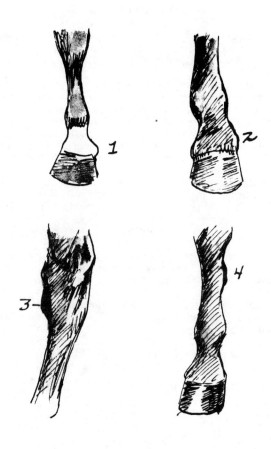

PLATE XVIII

Fig. 1, Sidebone. Fig. 2, Ringbone. Fig. 3,
Spavin. Fig. 4, Splint.

The "spavin test" is sometimes useful in diagnosing spavin lameness. It consists in keeping the hock joint flexed for one or two minutes and then trotting the horse. If a spavin exists lameness is very marked.

Treatment. The treatment of bone spavin is the same as that prescribed for ringbone.

SPLINTS

Splints are bony enlargements, usually situated between the inner splint bone and the cannon bone, at their upper third. They occasionally occur on the outside of the hind leg.

Causes. Faulty action or faulty conformation causing unequal distribution of pressure in the knee may throw an excessive load on the inner small metacarpal and cause rupture of the tissue affixing the small to the large metacarpal. The irritation produces growth of bone.

Symptoms. Soreness may or may not be present; when the splint is painful the horse is lame.

Treatment. If there is lameness give the animal absolute rest and apply a blister composed as follows: Biniodide of mercury 1 dram, cosmoline 5 drams. Repeat in ten days if necessary.

DETECTION OF LAMENESS

Severe lameness is readily recognized, even when the animal is at rest. Distinct symptoms, such as pointing or frequent raising of the affected limb, are noticed, the animal's instinct leading him to place the affected part in a position to relieve the pain.

In making an examination for lameness, the animal, having free use of his head, should be led at a slow trot toward and from the observer. Too short a hold on the halter shank will prevent free play of all the muscles concerned in locomotion.

If lame in one fore leg, the right one for instance, the head will nod (drop) more or less when he steps on the left fore leg, while the head jerks up at the moment the right leg (the lame one) is placed upon the ground. Hence, the head of the lame animal always nods when the sound leg is planted.

Should there be lameness in both fore legs the action is stilty (stiff); the natural, elastic stride is wanting; the steps are shortened, and the feet kept close to the ground. Almost invariably the hind legs are picked up higher than normally; the shoulders appear stiff and the head is carried rather high, while the lumbar region is arched.

Lameness behind is detected by trotting the horse from the observer, the croup being the essential part to be watched, since it drops with the sound leg and rises with the lame one.

If lame in both hind legs, the stride is shortened and awkward; the fore legs are kept back of the vertical line, and are apt to be raised higher than usual, while the head is lowered. Backing is difficult; it is almost impossible to keep the animal at a trot when he is lame in more than one leg.

Horses lame in both fore or both hind legs show a waddling gait behind, often mistaken for lameness originating in the lumbar region. This peculiar motion is simply due to the fact that the hind legs are unduly advanced under the body for their own relief or that of the front legs. Close attention is to be paid to the animal's action as he turns while being trotted to and from the observer, as at this moment –

that is, while he turns — any hitch becomes visible; as, for instance, spavin or stringhalt lameness.

Always place the lame leg in its natural position and inspect the various parts of the leg both with the hand and eye, comparing them always with the sound leg to find anatomical changes.

In all cases examine the foot thoroughly and carefully, removing the shoe if necessary. Heat, pain, and swelling are always guides in the diagnosis of lameness.

All lameness is divided into two classes: *Swinging-leg* lameness, which is shown by a shortened stride and more or less dragging of the leg; and *supporting-leg* lameness, which shows itself when the leg supports the weight of the body. The former is shown in diseased condition of the muscles. The latter is shown in disease of bone, tendons, ligaments, and the hoof.

CHAPTER XII

AGE BY THE TEETH

By their growth, changes, form, and wear, the teeth of the horse furnish a very reliable guide to determine the animal's age. In the adult animal they number from 36 in the female to 40 in the male, and are classed according to their location, form, and function, as *incisors, canines,* and *molars.*

The incisors, or *cutters,* occupy the front part of the mouth. They are 12 in number, 6 in the upper jaw and 6 in the lower. In each jaw there are 2 central, 2 lateral, and 2 corner incisors.

The canines, or *tushes,* occupy the front part of the interdental space. The tushes are usually absent in the mare, or, if present, are very small. They are 4 in number, 2 in each jaw.

The molars, or *grinders,* occupy the back part of the mouth. They are twenty-four in number, 6 on each side of each jaw. Naming from front to rear they are designated first, second, third, etc. Quite frequently supplementary molars, called "wolf teeth," are present. If so, they appear directly in front of the first molar, in the upper jaw, and very rarely in the lower jaw.

Like other animals, the horse is provided with two sets of teeth, temporary and permanent. The temporary, or milk teeth, are those of the first growth or dentition. They are 24 in number, 12 incisors and the first, second, and third molars. They are all up and in wear when the colt is about 11 months old. Each of them is ultimately shed and replaced by a permanent tooth. The first shedding takes place at 2½ and the last is completed at 4½ years of age. The first permanent tooth to show itself, however, is the fourth molar, which appears at about the age of 1 year.

The permanent incisor differs in appearance from the temporary one by being larger, longer, darker, or more yellowish in color, and by having a well-marked groove down the anterior or front face of the crown. It does not have the constricted neck which is characteristic of the milk tooth.

The three principal tooth substances are called *dentine, enamel,* and *cement.* The dentine composes the main body of the tooth. It is protected by a covering of enamel, which is very white in color and is the hardest of all animal substances. The cement is a yellowish colored bony material. It also forms a protective covering for the tooth, being spread in a thin layer over the surface of the enamel. This cement gives the permanent tooth the color which distinguishes it from the milk tooth. By the time the animal is 7 or 8 years of age, this substance, through constant rubbing by the lips and washing with saliva, has been worn from the enamel, and the teeth consequently appear much whiter than they did when the animal was but 5 or 6.

The grinding surface of the tooth is called the *table.* In the new unworn tooth this is irregular and is covered with enamel. The *infundibulum* is the infolding of the enamel on the table of the tooth. This forms in the incisors a cavity, the bottom of which is filled with cement to a depth which varies in different animals. The unfilled portion of this cavity forms what is called the *cup.* The cups are deeper in the upper incisors than they are in the lower ones. They soon become stained by the food juices so that they appear very black in color. Ordinarily after a lower incisor has been in wear for three years its table surface has been worn down to the cement filling and the blackened cup cavity has disappeared. It is often difficult for the inexperienced observer to determine when the cup has actually disappeared. He expects to see the table surface perfectly level and of uniform color, whereas the enamel being so much harder than either the dentine or the cement, stands in relief on the table surface, and envelops a very shallow and sometimes slightly stained depression (of cement) for several years after the black cup cavity is considered to have disappeared. The enamel of the infundibulum persists in the lowers usually until the animal is about 15 and in the uppers until he is about 18 years of age. Standing in relief on the table surface as it does, this enamel is frequently termed "the enamel island."

In the center of the tooth, and extending almost its entire length, is the *pulp cavity*, a channel, which in life is filled with a fleshy tissue or pulp through the medium of which the tooth derives its nourishment. As the tooth is worn off with age the outer extremity of the sensitive pulp, which would otherwise become exposed, is changed into a yellowish colored ivory-like substance that completely fills and closes the cavity. Hence, when the tooth has worn down to the pulp cavity, the latter appears on the table surface (just in front of the remains of the cup) as a yellowish colored mark called the *dental star*. This usually makes its appearance when the animal is 8 years old, although in very hard teeth it is often not apparent until about 11.

Depending upon the hardness of the dentine and the character of the food, the teeth wear away at the rate of about one-twelfth of an inch per year. As an incisor is not of uniform shape or size from its crown to its root, it is at once apparent that wear will continually change the form of its table surface.

In the young mouth the tables of the incisors are elongated from side to side, while in the old mouth they are elongated from front to rear. The intermediate forms through which they successively pass are oval, round, and triangular. Roughly speaking, the incisors are oval from 7 till 9 (centrals at 7, laterals at 8, and corners at 9), round from 10 till 13, triangular from 14 till 17, and elongated from front to rear at 18 or 19.

In the young animal, while the teeth are still unworn to any extent, the upper and lower incisors meet in such a way that they appear as an evenly rounded arch. This arch, however, gradually changes as the teeth wear away, until in age it has become very angular or pointed.

In examining the mouth of the horse to determine his age, three features of the incisor teeth are studied: First, the angle at which the uppers and lowers meet; second, the character and color of their crown faces, and, third, the shape and appearance of the tables.

To obtain the best view of the mouth, grasp the upper lip firmly with the right hand, and place the left in the interdental space from the right side, using the thumb to depress the lower lip, and the back of the hand to press the tongue upward and backward. In this way the right hand serves as a twitch to hold the horse, while the left one uncovers the lower incisors.

As has already been stated, the temporary teeth are all up and in wear at about the age of 11 months. Between the ages of 1 and 2 the incisors remain the same in their arrangement, but begin to show the effects of wear.

At 2 the mouth presents very much the same appearance as it does at 5, the difference being that the incisors are *temporary* in the former and permanent in the latter, and that the 2-year-old has but *five molars* on the side of each jaw, while the 5-year-old has all *six*. This is the *only case* in which the molars might render assistance in the determination of the age. At about the age of 2½ years the temporary centrals are pushed out by permanent ones. The uppers are usually shed a few weeks before the lowers. After these teeth make their appearance, and until they are up and in wear, the horse is rising, that is approaching, 3.

At 3 the colt has two permanent incisors (the centrals) and four temporary ones (the laterals and corners) in each jaw. The centrals are up and in wear; that is, they are on a level with the temporary teeth. The permanent centrals are seen to be darker or more yellowish in color than their neighbors, and to have a well-marked groove down their front face. Another important observation to make is the appearance of the cups. In either the temporary or the permanent full mouth, the centrals, having been in wear for the longest period of time, show the shallowest cups, while in the 3-year-old mouth the new centrals, having been in wear for the shortest period of time, show the largest, deepest, and blackest ones. The colt is said to be 3 years past when the permanent centrals show wear on both their front and rear borders. At about the age of 3½ years the temporary laterals are shed, and until their permanent successors are up and in wear the colt is rising 4.

At 4 the colt has four permanent incisors (the centrals and laterals) and two temporary ones (the corners) in each jaw. The laterals are worn on both their front and rear borders, and the cups of the lower centrals, having been in wear for one year and being about one-third gone, show smaller than the cups of the laterals. At this age the contrast between the large permanent incisors and the small temporary corners is very striking. The colt is about 4½ years old when the corners begin to shed. At about this time the mouth of the male begins to show the tushes. After the temporary corners have all been shed, and until the four permanent corners are in contact, the colt is rising 5.

At 5 the mouth is full. All the incisors are now permanent, and in each jaw they have all reached the same level. The front borders of the corners are in wear but the rear borders are not yet up. The cuts of the centrals, having been in wear for two years, are about two-thirds gone, while those of the laterals, having been in wear for one year, are about one-third gone. Usually the rear borders of the corners come up and in the wear while the animal is between 5 and 6 years old, but sometimes they do not come up as they should, and such a condition constitutes what is known as a *shell mouth.* This condition may cause an 8-year-old animal to be mistaken for a 6-year-old.

At 6 the cup cavities are worn entirely out of the centrals, two-thirds out of the laterals, and one-third out of the corners. At 6 past, a notch begins to form on the outer border of the upper corners.

At 7 the cups are gone from the centrals and the laterals, and the notch which began forming at 6 past on the upper corners is now well marked. The enamel is now beginning to lose its cement covering, with the result that the teeth are showing whiter than they did when the animal was 6. The tables of the centrals are becoming oval in form.

At 8 the blackened cups have usually disappeared from all of the lower incisors, although in some cases those of the corners persist for a year or two longer. The notch in the upper corners is hardly as prominent at this age as it was at 7 because, on account of wear, the angle of meeting is now beginning to change, and the upper corners in consequence are finding a greater grinding surface on the lower ones. In some cases the dental star may now be detected between the enamel island and the front border of the tooth in the central incisors. It appears in the form of a yellowish transverse line.

After the age of 6 wear alone, by changing the form and appearance of the table surfaces and the angle at which the uppers and lowers meet, furnishes the indications of age; and as the wear varies with the hardness of the teeth and the character of the food, it is at once apparent that no two cases will be exactly the same. Hence, after the animal is 8 years old the age indications have become unreliable. From now on with the passing of each year they become less and less reliable. After the twelfth year there is but little probability of judging the age accurately.

On an average, it is found that the cups of the upper incisors are worn out in the centrals at the age of ten.

At 15 in most cases the enamel island has disappeared from the lowers, and the dental star has become distinct and round in the center of the tables. The enamel island persists in the uppers usually until the animal is about 18.

After 20 the horse is considered to have reached the limit of his life. The characters then presented by the teeth are those of extreme age. The table surfaces are elongated from front to rear. Sometimes the crowns are very long and extend almost in prolongation of the jaws. Sometimes they are very short and are worn down to a level with the gums. The crowns now appear to converge toward the median line, whereas in youth they appeared straight or slightly divergent.

Many deceptions may be practiced or many conditions may exist which render the determination of the age very difficult. Some dishonest dealers and breeders resort to pulling the milk teeth a few months before they would fall, thereby hastening the appearance of the permanent ones and giving the mouth an older appearance. Sometimes the notches in the upper corners are rasped away to make the 7-year-old mouth look younger. *"Bishoping"* is another form of deception that is sometimes practiced. This is done to make an old mouth appear young. New cups are drilled in the old teeth, and these cups are then stained black by some artificial means. This practice, however, should never deceive the close observer because the ring of enamel, which is always present around the natural cup, can not be reproduced in the bishoped mouth. Moreover the teeth will show by the angle at which they meet and by the form of their table surfaces that the mouth is too old for cups to be present.

Horses with parrot or overshot mouths, and horses in the habit of cribbing, subject their teeth to unnatural wear, which renders the determination of their age very difficult.

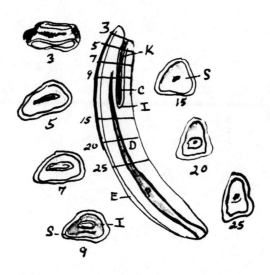

PLATE XIX

Longitudinal Section of left central lower incisor and cross sections of same tooth showing table surfaces as they appear at the ages of 3, 5, 7, 9, 15, 20 and 25 years.

C, Cement	D, Dentine	E, Enamel
I, Infundibulum	K, Cup	P, Pulp Cavity
	S, Star	

CHAPTER XIII

TROPICAL DISEASES

SURRA

This disease is caused by the *Trypanasoma Evansi,* an organism which is a low form of animal life and is found in the blood of affected animals. It attacks and destroys the red blood cells, causing rapid loss of flesh and, sooner or later, death. It is claimed by some authorities that the disease originates from the use of water and grass from low lands.

Symptoms. Variable temperature, ranging from normal to 102° and even to 106° F.; dullness; lack of vigor; sometimes swelling of the submaxillary lymph glands; thin, watery discharge from the nostrils; swelling of the sheath and legs, more frequently the hind ones, and swelling along the belly; these swellings pit on pressure. The mucous membrane of the eye, especially of the haw, shows dark-red spots (petechial spots); the urine is highly colored and is usually passed in large quantities; the bowels are constipated in the early stage and profuse diarrhea occurs later. In chronic cases paralysis of the hind extremities takes place, the animal staggering when moved. The paralysis may later become complete and the horse will be unable to rise. In the acute type of the disease the animal dies in twelve or fifteen days, while in the chronic case he may linger for one or two months. The diagnosis is complete only when a microscopic examination of the blood discloses the parasite. As a rule, the parasite is seen only when the temperature is considerably elevated.

Surra is always fatal, and as the danger to other animals is great on account of its highly contagious nature, all animals that have been proved to have the parasite in the blood should be removed at once from contact with healthy stock and destroyed. The carcasses should be saturated with oil and burned. Measures to prevent the spread of the disease should always be enforced. When in a district infested with surra the temperature of horses should be taken regularly every two or three days. Any animal showing, without a known cause, a temperature of 102° F. should be isolated, and thereafter blood examinations should be made and temperatures taken daily. As flies are known to be carriers of the surra parasite, great care should be exercised to remove and avoid any breeding places for these pests. If stables could be screened in would be a great advantage in surra outbreaks.

EPIZOOTIC OR ULCERATIVE LYMPHANGITIS

This peculiar tropical disease closely resembles glanders of the farcy form, so much so that the two might be easily confused by a person uninformed on tropical diseases. In observing epizootic lymphangitis the high fever and sudden loss of flesh and vigor are not seen as in tropical glanders.

The disease in the early stage responds to treatment, but often requires months to effect a cure. It is caused by a fungus, called *cryptococcus,* and is contagious.

Symptoms. Small bunches or nodules, the size of a half dollar, may appear upon the skin of any part of the body; there may be one or many. They often appear in chains along the course of the lymphatics; they may spread around an infected area into an irregular patch, apparently not following the lymphatics; again, the disease may start with a hard, painful swelling in the region of the chest or

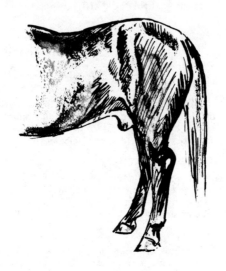

PLATE XIXa.

Surra: Characteristic swellings.

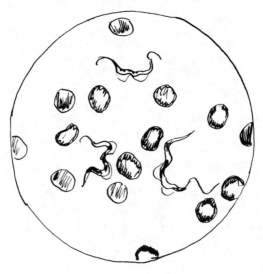

PLATE XX

Surra parasite.

90

shoulder, or between the forelegs, the swelling later softening in spits and forming the small abscesses.

Ordinarily, the nodules soon soften and break upon the surface; if not, they should be opened; in either case they end in the typical ulcers of the disease. The small bunches or abscesses, when opened, contain a white, creamy pus; they do not respond readily to ordinary healing methods and persist after the most heroic measures have been adopted. In cases of long standing the ulcerations may extend over the greater part of the body, the limbs especially being covered with sores; there is usually great enlargement and thickening of the legs and the patient becomes badly emaciated (poor in flesh). In the ordinary case, however, the animal does not lose flesh and does not carry any marked fever.

Treatment. The treatment consists in opening the ulcers freely with a knife or cautery point heated to white heat, or, better still, if they are not too numerous, in dissecting them out entirely without opening the abscess wall.

The dressings must be of a caustic nature, so as to destroy the cause of the disease; for instance, alcohol 4 ounces, salicylic acid 1 ounce, bichloride of mercury 2 drams; alternate this with a dressing made of equal parts of olive oil and creolin, or one made of tincture of iodine 2 ounces and tincture of iron 2 ounces. Apply any of these dressings once daily and then use a dusting powder made of equal parts of iodoform and tannic acid.

Care should be exercised to isolate the diseased animals and to thoroughly disinfect combs, brushes, blankets, halters, and such articles as may have come in contact with the diseased parts; for this purpose use a 1 to 20 solution of creolin or of carbolic acid.

DHOBIE ITCH

This is a very troublesome skin disease peculiar to the Tropics. It is contagious and caused by a fungus.

Symptoms. – Itching, the animal rubbing against the posts and sides of the stall; small eruptions of the skin, which spread rapidly and discharge a thin, watery secretion, crusts forming over the sores; the hair falls out and the skin becomes thickened on account of the irritation. Often the skin of a large part of the surface of the body becomes infected with these sores, and ordinary healing washes have no beneficial action. The treatment, like that of epizootic lymphangitis, should be prompt and energetic, and, since both diseases are caused by a fungus, should be similar in nature.

One of the most valuable remedies is made of equal parts of olive oil and creolin, which should be applied once daily after thoroughly washing the sores and removing the scabs. A mixture of alcohol 6 ounces and salicylic acid 1 ounce is of value and is applied daily. In the absence of alcohol, sulphuric ether may be substituted. Tincture of iodine often effects a cure. If the case is persistent, cauterize the parts with pure carbolic acid and then apply alcohol after the acid has been on one minute. After cauterizing use the olive oil and creolin dressing daily.

On account of its contagious nature, all animals suffering from this disease should be isolated, and brushes, combs, blankets, etc., should be thoroughly disinfected with creolin or carbolic acid solution.

The common diseases of temperate countries assume a more aggravated form in the Tropics. Infectious diseases are more fatal and infected wounds heal more slowly. This is due to the lower vitality of the animal and to the hot and moist climate, which favors germ growth. Pneumonia is almost always fatal in the Philippines. Canker and thrush are found in the most aggravated type. Periodic ophthalmia is very prevalent, resulting in many animals becoming blind. Heatstroke is a frequent occurrence, on account of the excessive heat and moisture, and is fatal in the majority of cases. The temperature in heatstroke frequently rises to 110° to 113° F. Glanders, which is very common, runs a rapid and fatal course. American horses rarely suffer from the chronic form of the disease often manifested in cooler climates.

In the Tropics a careful daily inspection of the horses should be made and the temperature of every animal should be taken at least once a week. Any animal with a suspicious discharge from the nose or with sores upon the body indicating farcy buds and any animal showing a rise of 2 degrees above normal temperature should be isolated and kept under observation by a veterinarian. In case of an outbreak, temperatures should be taken daily. Normal temperature in the Tropics is usually about 1 degree higher than in a cool climate, and it may rise as much as 4 degrees with exercise of a moderate nature. These facts should be taken into consideration in recording temperatures.

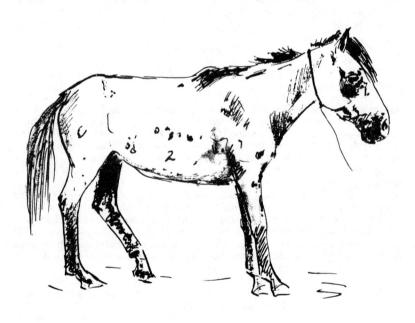

PLATE XXI

Chronic epizootic lymphangitis (tropical).

CHAPTER XIV

MEDICINES; THEIR ACTION AND USES

Antiseptics. Remedies which arrest putrefaction. They kill or prevent the development of those bacteria which produce decomposition.
Examples: Corros, sub., carbolic acid, creolin.

Disinfectants. Destroy the specific poisons of communicable diseases by killing those germs which produce disease.
Examples: Lime, sulphur gas, etc.

Deodorants. Disguise or destroy odors.
Examples: Iron sulphate, carbolic acid, etc.

Rubefacients. Cause redness of the skin.
Examples: Alcohol, turpentine, etc.

Vesicants. Cause a discharge of serum from the skin.
Example: Cantharides.

Stomachics. Promote digestion.
Examples: Gentian, ginger, etc.

Vermicides. Kill worms.
Examples: Turpentine, iron sulphate, etc.

Vermifuges. Remove intestinal worms by purgation.

Parasiticides. Destroy parasites.
Examples: Carbolic acid, creolin, etc.

Purgatives. Evacuate the bowels.
Example: Aloes.

Laxatives. Mild purgatives.
Examples: Bran mash, small dose of linseed oil.

Cholagogues. Promote secretion of bile.
Examples: Aloes, calomel.

Diaphoretics. Increase perspiration.
Examples: Ethers. Same action produced mechanically by warm clothing.

Diuretics. Increase secretion of urine.
Examples: Potass, nit., turpentine.

Tonics. Gradually but permanently improve appetite and increase vigor.
Examples: Quinine, iron, gentian, etc.

Anesthetics. Produce loss of consciousness.
Example: Chloroform.

Styptics. Check hemorrhage.
Example: Tincture of iron.

Caustics. Destroy tissue by burning.
Examples: Lunar caustic, copper sulphate, etc.

Expectorants. Act upon the mucous membrane of the respiratory organs and cause an expulsion of their secretions.
Example: Chloride of ammonia.

Stimulants. Promptly but temporarily increase nervous vigor, thus increasing action of the heart and other functions.
Examples: Alcohol, ammonia, ether.

Alteratives. Correct morbid conditions without causing marked physiological effects.
Examples: Iodide of potassium, potassium nitrate.

Astringents. Contract living tissues.
Examples: Alum, zinc sulphate, tannic acid.

Sedatives. Depress (slow) the nervous system.
Examples: Potas, bromide.

Anodynes. Relieve pain by diminishing the excitability of nerves and nerve centers.
Examples: Opium, belladonna.

Antispasmodics. Prevent or remove spasmodic contractions of voluntary or involuntary muscles.
Examples: Belladonna, sulphuric ether.

Carminatives. Aid in the expulsion of gas from the intestines by increasing natural movement, stimulating circulation, etc.
Examples: Capsicum, ginger, aromatic spts. ammonia, sulphuric ether, etc.

Febrifuges or antipyretics. Agents which reduce high temperature of the blood; reduce fever.
Examples: Acetanilid, cold water.

VETERINARY MEDICINES

Acetanilid. Is a febrifuge and antiseptic. Used internally to lower fever in doses of from 1 to 4 drams. Used externally as an antiseptic in the form of a dry dressing.

Acid, arsenious (arsenic). Is an irritant, corrosive, poison, given internally in doses of from 1 to 6 grains as a digestive tonic, and for skin diseases, usually in combination with iron sulphate and gentian. Externally it is used to remove warts, in the form of an ointment, 1 part of arsenic to 8 or 10 of lard.

Acid, boracic. Action, antiseptic; a saturated solution is very useful in conjunctivitis. With oxide of zinc it makes a very nice dressing for abrasions, scratches, etc.

Acid, carbolic. A valuable antiseptic and disinfectant. A 1 to 20 solution makes a very good wash for all wounds. A very good prescription for local use is the following:

> Carbolic acid, 6 drams.
> Glycerin, 1½ ounces.
> Water to make 1 pint.

Acid, salicylic. A useful antiseptic; a saturated solution of salicylic acid in alcohol is a good dressing for indolent sores and ulcers.
Salicylic acid dusted upon a wound will remove the granulations of proud flesh.

Acid, tannic. An astringent and antiseptic. It is given internally in diarrhea and dysentery. Dose, 30 grains to 1 dram.
The following prescription may be used:

> Acid, tannic, ½ to 1 dram.
> Opium, powdered, ½ to 1 dram.

Make into one ball and repeat every two hours until the diarrhea is checked.
Tannic acid is an excellent remedy, used in the form of a saturated solution (with witchhazel water), for hardening tender shoulders.

Aconite. Is a dangerous poison and should not be used internally, but locally. Mixed with other drugs it makes a good anodyne liniment.

> Aconite, 2 ounces.
> Alcohol, 5 ounces.
> Opium, tincture, 4 ounces.
> Witchhazel, distilled, 5 ounces.

Mix, and apply several times daily.

Alcohol. Stimulant. Given for weak heart in debilitating diseases, such as lung troubles, etc. Dose, 2 to 4 ounces in 1 pint of water, and repeated every four to six hours, as required.
It is useful in the formation of liniments.

Aloes, Barbados. Is the general purgative for the horse. Dose, 6 to 8 drams.

> Aloes, Barbados, 6 to 8 drams.
> Ginger, 1 dram.

Make into a ball and give upon an empty stomach.

The "cathartic capsule," to be supplied, will take the place of aloes. It will contain aloin, strychnine, ginger, and calomel.

A purgative should never be given in diseases of the respiratory system.

It generally takes about twenty-four hours to operate.

Alum. Astringent. It is useful as a wash for sore mouths; used in the strength of ½ ounce to 1 quart of water. Externally it is a valuable remedy in the treatment of thrush. Burnt alum is useful for the removal of proud flesh.

Ammonia, aromatic spirits of. Stimulant and carminative. A very useful remedy in the treatment of colics, and exhaustion. Dose, 1 to 3 ounces, well diluted.

Ammonia, solution of. Used externally only, in combination with other drugs, as a stimulating liniment.

> Ammonia, solution of, 1 part.
> Turpentine, oil of, 1 part.
> Olive oil, 2 parts.

To be well shaken before using. It is an excellent external application for sore throat.

Ammonia, chloride of. Used in all cases where an expectorant is indicated, such as diseases of the respiratory system. Dose, 1 to 4 drams. For catarrhal diseases it is usually combined with quinine and nitrate of potash, prepared in the following manner:

> Ammonia, chloride of, 3 ounces.
> Quinine sulphate, 6 drams.
> Nitrate of potash, 3 ounces.

Make into twelve powders and give one every three or four hours.

Belladonna, fluid extract. Antispasmodic and anodyne. Used in cases of colic in conjunction with other medicines. Dose, 1 to 2 drams.

When applied to the eyes it dilates the pupil and soothes the irritated membrane. Generally used in combination with sulphate of zinc or boracicacid solutions.

A very useful wash for the treatment of conjunctivitis is made as follows:

> Sulphate of zinc, 20 grains.
> Belladonna, fld. ext., 1 dram.
> Water, 3½ ounces.

Apply twice a day.

Camphor, gum. Antispasmodic and antiseptic. Dose, 1 to 2 drams. A very good remedy for diarrhea is made as follows:

> Camphor, gum, 1 dram.
> Opium, powdered, 1 dram.

Make into a ball; give, and repeat every two hours until relief is afforded.

Externally it is useful for sprains, combined with other medicines, forming what is known as the soap liniment.

> Castile soap, 10 parts.
> Camphor, 5 parts.
> Alcohol, 70 parts.
> Water, 15 parts.

To be used only externally as a mild, stimulating, anodyne liniment.

A useful dressing for wounds is made of gum camphor, 8 ounces, carbolic acid, 3 ounces. This is especially valuable in fly time.

Cannabis indica (Indian hemp). Antispasmodic and anodyne. Its main use is in colic, as it relieves pain without causing constipation. Dose, 2 to 4 drams.

> Cannabis indica, 2 to 4 drams.
> Ammonia, aromatic spirits, 1 ounce.
> Water, 1 pint.

Give at one dose and repeat in three-quarters of an hour if necessary. This is an excellent remedy for colic.

Cantharides, powdered (Spanish fly). Used only for its blistering effect. Prepare by rubbing the cantharides and cosmoline together (1 to 5 or 6) with a spatula on a piece of glass.

Capsicum (cayenne pepper). Stomachic and carminative. Given internally in combination with gentian and ginger in mild cases of indigestion attended with flatulency. Dose, ½ to 1 dram.

Charcoal. A mild antiseptic and deodorant. It is very good mixed with poultices, especially for wounds and sores that have a foul odor. It may be dusted on the surface of foul sores and will soon destroy the odor. Internally it is given in doses of 2 to 4 drams, and is useful in chronic indigestion and diarrhea.

Copper sulphate (blue vitriol, bluestone). A caustic, tonic, vermicide, and astringent. Used principally as a caustic for thrush and canker. A good remedy for thrush or canker is equal parts of sulphate of copper (powdered), sulphate of zinc, and sulphate of iron: *"The three sulphates."* This powder can be applied two or three times daily. Used also internally as a tonic in chronic nasal catarrh. Dose, 1 to 2 drams.

Collodion. When painted over wounds it forms an air-tight coating and in small wounds keeps the edges in a fixed position and promotes healing. Especially valuable when applied to punctured wounds of joints.

Chloroform. Antispasmodic, stimulant, and anodyne. Useful in colics. Dose, 1 to 2 drams, well diluted. It may be added to anodyne liniments. When inhaled, it acts as an anesthetic.

Cosmoline. A by-product of petroleum. Used as a base for ointments. It is also valuable to apply upon the skin, when wound secretions are abundant to prevent dropping out of the hair.

Creolin. A nonpoisonous, nonirritating antiseptic and parasiticide. It is one of the best medicines that we have, not only as a valuable application for all wounds, but to destroy all parasites with which the animal may become infested.
Used in solution or ointment in a strength of 1 to 50 or 1 to 20. For mange it is used in a 1 to 10 solution.

Digitalis, fluid extract of. A very dangerous poison, and should not be administered internally. A valuable diuretic when applied over the kidneys and well rubbed in.

Ether, nitrous, spirits of (sweet spirits of niter). Stimulant, antispasmodic, diuretic, and diaphoretic. Dose, 1 to 2 ounces.
A very useful stimulant in all cases of weakness of the heart action. For its stimulating and antispasmodic actions it is given in colics combined with belladonna or cannabis indica.

Ether, sulphuric. Stimulant, antispasmodic, and carminative. Dose, 1 to 2 ounces, well diluted.
Combined with belladonna or cannabis indica its antispasmodic action is increased.

Fenugreek. Aromatic and stomachic. Sometimes combined with tonics to disguise their odors. Dose, 1 ounce.

Flaxseed meal. Used for poultices.

Gentian. Stomachic and bitter tonic. It improves the appetite and general tone. Dose, ½ to 1 ounce.

Ginger. Stomachic and carminative. Combined with purgatives it diminishes their tendency to gripe, and also somewhat hastens their action. Dose, ½ to 1 ounce.

Glycerin. Used as a base in the same manner as cosmoline. Useful, combined with equal parts of iodine, in the treatment of grease.

Iodine. Given internally in diabetes insipidus. Dose, 20 grains to 1 dram, to be repeated three times daily until the quantity of urine is lessened. Best given made into a ball with flaxseed meal.

Externally it is used for the removal of swellings, curbs, enlarged tendons, etc. It is also a useful stimulant for indolent sores and ulcers. A good solution for external use is made as follows:

> Iodine, 1 ounce.
> Iodide of potassium, 3 ounces.
> Water, 1 pint.

To be applied several times daily.

Tincture of iodine is made of iodine, 1 ounce; alcohol, 1 pint.

Iodoform. Antiseptic. Used externally as a dry dressing, either alone or combined with other drugs, such as boracic acid, acetanilid, etc.

Iron, tincture of the chloride of. A valuable tonic, building up the system and enriching the blood. Useful in purpura and in convalescence after all debilitating diseases. Dose, 1 to 2 ounces, well diluted.

Used externally as an astringent and styptic in serious hemorrhages. A small piece of cotton saturated with it and applied to the bleeding part is the proper mode of application.

Iron, sulphate of (Ferrisulphate). Tonic and vermicide. It increases the appetite and builds up the system. Dose, ½ to 1 dram. Frequently combined with nux vomica, etc.

Lanolin. Used as a base for ointments in the same manner as cosmoline.

Lead, acetate of. Astringent and a valuable remedy for relieving local pain. Used externally to cool and relieve sprains, inflamed tendons and joints, and to relieve itching skin diseases.

The white lotion is made as follows:

> Acetate of lead, 1 ounce.
> Sulphate of zinc, 1 ounce.
> Water, 1 quart.

Shake well and apply several times daily.

The lotion is a very valuable remedy for the relief of all external diseases accompanied by heat and swelling; also an excellent dressing for wounds.

Lime, chloride of. This is the best disinfectant that we have. Four ounces to 1 gallon of water is the proper strength. This solution should be used as a wash for the disinfection of stables. A small portion of chloride of lime placed around the stables will destroy the odor arising from decomposed urine.

Lunar caustic. Used for the removal of warts and proud flesh. Four grains to 1 ounce of water make a good application for the removal of the cloudiness remaining after an attack of ophthalmia.

Mercury, bichloride of (corrosive sublimate; antiseptic tablets). Dissolved in water this is the most energetic antiseptic; 1 to 1,000 solution is the proper strength to use in the treatment of all wounds. Two tablets to a quart of water give this strength; if the bichloride is in bulk, use 15 grains to a quart of water, and add 15 grains of chloride of ammonia to insure complete dissolution.

Mercury, mild chloride (calomel). Internally, a cholagogue. Dose, ½ to 2 drams. It is not used alone, but is combined with aloes.

> Calomel, 1 dram.
> Barbados aloes, 4 drams.
> Ginger, 1 dram.
> Water to make a ball.

Externally, antiseptic and drying. Used in the treatment of ulcers and thrush.

Mercury, biniodide. Used as a blister; its effects are very penetrating. Used principally in the treatment of spavins, splints, sidebones, ringbones, and all bony enlargements.

> Biniodide of mercury, 1 part.
> Cosmoline, 5 to 6 parts.

Mix and rub together thoroughly.
Apply with friction for at least ten minutes.

Nux vomica, powdered. A nerve stimulant and tonic. Dose, ½ to 1 dram. It is a very useful tonic in building up the tone of the system in convalescence from debilitating diseases and general lack of vitality. Generally given in combination with gentian, iron, and other tonics.

Oil, linseed. Laxative (mild purgative). Dose, ½ to 1 quart. Do not use boiled oil.

Oil, olive. Generally used as a vehicle in making liniments and oily solutions.

Oil of tar (pine tar). Useful for plugging holes and cavities in the hoof after all suppuration has ceased.

Oil of turpentine. Diuretic, stimulant, antispasmodic, vermicide, and expectorant. Dose, 1 to 3 ounces diluted with oil.
Externally it is used in the formation of liniments (see Solution of Ammonia).

Opium, tincture of (laudanum). Anodyne. antispasmodic. Checks secretion of mucus membrane. On account of these properties it is a valuable remedy in diarrhea and dysentery.

Very useful in the treatment of all abdominal pain where there are no symptoms of constipation, but as a rule belladonna and cannabis indica are preferable. Dose, 1 to 2 ounces.

Externally, opium tincture is used to relieve pain of sprains and bruises.

A very good anodyne lotion is made as follows:

Opium tincture, 4 ounces.
Acetate of lead, 2 ounces.
Water to make 1 quart.

Apply every few hours.

Opium, powdered. Not used externally. It is used internally for the same purpose as the tincture. Dose, ½ to 2 drams.

Potassium bromide. Nerve sedative. Dose, ½ to 2 ounces. In tetanus this medicine can be given in large doses.

Potassium nitrate (saltpeter). Alterative, febrifuge, and diuretic. Dose, 1 to 4 drams. In the treatment of laminitis the dose is 2 to 4 ounces, repeated three times a day. Externally it makes a good cooling lotion:

Nitrate potassium (saltpeter), 5 ounces.
Chloride of ammonia, 5 ounces.
Water, 16 ounces.

Mix and keep the affected parts saturatèd with this lotion.

Internally, saltpeter is a most excellent medicine in the treatment of catarrhal and febrile diseases. It is also useful in the treatment of swollen legs.

Potassium iodide. Alterative, diuretic, and expectorant. Dose, 2 to 4 drams. It is given to promote absorption of enlargements, such as enlarged glands in lymphangitis, and in partial paralysis resulting from injury to the brain or spinal cord.

For such purposes full doses are given twice a day for two weeks.

Potassium permanganate. Antiseptic, disinfectant, and deodorant. Useful for the removal of foul odors arising from unhealthy wounds; also for cleaning hands and instruments. From 1 to 4 drams, water 1 pint, is the proper strength of the solution for use.

Quinine, sulphate of. Tonic, stomachic, antiseptic, and mild febrifuge. Dose, ½ to 1 dram, repeated three times a day. It is given in all febrile and debilitating diseases. Combined with sulphate of iron it is very useful in purpura. In influenza and pneumonia it is generally combined with gentian and nitrate of potash, made into powders in the following proportions:

Quinine sulphate, 1 ounce.
Gentian, 3 ounces.

Make twelve powders and give three times a day.

Salol. Antiseptic. Used internally and externally for its antiseptic properties. Dose, 2 to 4 drams.

Sodium bicarbonate. Carminative, stomachic, relieves acidity of the stomach. Dose, 1 to 2 drams. This is an excellent medicine in chronic indigestion and flatulency.

Sulphur. Parasiticide. This medicine may be used for the treatment of mange, but it is inferior to creolin or carbolic acid.

Witchhazel. A cooling astringent wash, very useful when combined with other medicines in the form of liniments or lotions.

Zinc sulphate. Externally it is much used as a caustic and astringent for wounds, foul ulcers, etc. It is an excellent remedy for the treatment of thrush and canker.

Sulphate of zinc
Sulphate of copper   Equal parts.
Sulphate of iron

Zinc oxide. Antiseptic and astringent. Used as a dry powder dusted on the wounds or can be made into an ointment with lanolin:

Zinc oxide, 1 part.
Lanolin, 6 parts.

Zinc chloride. An irritant and corrosive poison, never given internally. Externally it is applied as a stimulant, astringent, caustic, and parasiticide. It is also used as an antiseptic, disinfectant, and deodorant. From 2 to 4 drams to the pint of water are used for ordinary antiseptic purposes.

DOSES

Grouped according to amounts; for reference and for convenience in memorizing:

GRAINS

Arsenic 1 to 6   Iodine 20 to 60

DRAMS

½ to 1.   ½ to 1.
Capsicum; Iron sulphate; Nux vomica, powdered; Quinine sulphate; Tannic acid.

½ to 2.
Calomel; Opium, powdered.

1 to 2.
Bellandonna, fluid extract; Camphor, gum; Chloroform; Copper sulphate; Sodium bicarbonate.

1 to 4.
Acetanilid; Ammonia, chloride; Potassium, nitrate.

2 to 4.
Cannabis indica, fluid extract; Charcoal; Potassium iodide; Salol.

6 to 8.
Aloes.

OUNCES

½ to 1.
Gentian; Ginger.

1.
Fenugreek.

½ to 2.
Bromide of potassium.

1 to 2
Sulphuric ether; Sweet spirits of niter; Tinct. Chloride of iron; Tinct. Opium.

1 to 3.
Aromatic spirits of ammonia; Oil of turpentine.

2 to 4.
Alcohol; Potassium nitrate (in laminitis).

MELVIN POWERS SELF-IMPROVEMENT LIBRARY

ASTROLOGY

_____	ASTROLOGY: HOW TO CHART YOUR HOROSCOPE _Max Heindel_	5.00
_____	ASTROLOGY AND SEXUAL ANALYSIS _Morris C. Goodman_	5.00
_____	ASTROLOGY MADE EASY _Astarte_	3.00
_____	ASTROLOGY MADE PRACTICAL _Alexandra Kayhle_	3.00
_____	ASTROLOGY, ROMANCE, YOU AND THE STARS _Anthony Norvell_	4.00
_____	MY WORLD OF ASTROLOGY _Sydney Omarr_	7.00
_____	THOUGHT DIAL _Sydney Omarr_	4.00
_____	WHAT THE STARS REVEAL ABOUT THE MEN IN YOUR LIFE _Thelma White_	3.00

BRIDGE

_____	BRIDGE BIDDING MADE EASY _Edwin B. Kantar_	10.00
_____	BRIDGE CONVENTIONS _Edwin B. Kantar_	7.00
_____	BRIDGE HUMOR _Edwin B. Kantar_	5.00
_____	COMPETITIVE BIDDING IN MODERN BRIDGE _Edgar Kaplan_	4.00
_____	DEFENSIVE BRIDGE PLAY COMPLETE _Edwin B. Kantar_	15.00
_____	GAMESMAN BRIDGE—Play Better with Kantar _Edwin B. Kantar_	5.00
_____	HOW TO IMPROVE YOUR BRIDGE _Alfred Sheinwold_	5.00
_____	IMPROVING YOUR BIDDING SKILLS _Edwin B. Kantar_	4.00
_____	INTRODUCTION TO DECLARER'S PLAY _Edwin B. Kantar_	5.00
_____	INTRODUCTION TO DEFENDER'S PLAY _Edwin B. Kantar_	3.00
_____	KANTAR FOR THE DEFENSE _Edwin B. Kantar_	5.00
_____	KANTAR FOR THE DEFENSE VOLUME 2 _Edwin B. Kantar_	7.00
_____	SHORT CUT TO WINNING BRIDGE _Alfred Sheinwold_	3.00
_____	TEST YOUR BRIDGE PLAY _Edwin B. Kantar_	5.00
_____	VOLUME 2—TEST YOUR BRIDGE PLAY _Edwin B. Kantar_	5.00
_____	WINNING DECLARER PLAY _Dorothy Hayden Truscott_	5.00

BUSINESS, STUDY & REFERENCE

_____	CONVERSATION MADE EASY _Elliot Russell_	4.00
_____	EXAM SECRET _Dennis B. Jackson_	3.00
_____	FIX-IT BOOK _Arthur Symons_	2.00
_____	HOW TO DEVELOP A BETTER SPEAKING VOICE _M. Hellier_	4.00
_____	HOW TO SELF-PUBLISH YOUR BOOK & MAKE IT A BEST SELLER _Melvin Powers_	10.00
_____	INCREASE YOUR LEARNING POWER _Geoffrey A. Dudley_	3.00
_____	PRACTICAL GUIDE TO BETTER CONCENTRATION _Melvin Powers_	3.00
_____	PRACTICAL GUIDE TO PUBLIC SPEAKING _Maurice Forley_	5.00
_____	7 DAYS TO FASTER READING _William S. Schaill_	3.00
_____	SONGWRITERS' RHYMING DICTIONARY _Jane Shaw Whitfield_	6.00
_____	SPELLING MADE EASY _Lester D. Basch & Dr. Milton Finkelstein_	3.00
_____	STUDENT'S GUIDE TO BETTER GRADES _J. A. Rickard_	3.00
_____	TEST YOURSELF—Find Your Hidden Talent _Jack Shafer_	3.00
_____	YOUR WILL & WHAT TO DO ABOUT IT _Attorney Samuel G. Kling_	4.00

CALLIGRAPHY

_____	ADVANCED CALLIGRAPHY _Katherine Jeffares_	7.00
_____	CALLIGRAPHER'S REFERENCE BOOK _Anne Leptich & Jacque Evans_	7.00
_____	CALLIGRAPHY—The Art of Beautiful Writing _Katherine Jeffares_	7.00
_____	CALLIGRAPHY FOR FUN & PROFIT _Anne Leptich & Jacque Evans_	7.00
_____	CALLIGRAPHY MADE EASY _Tina Serafini_	7.00

CHESS & CHECKERS

_____	BEGINNER'S GUIDE TO WINNING CHESS _Fred Reinfeld_	5.00
_____	CHESS IN TEN EASY LESSONS _Larry Evans_	5.00
_____	CHESS MADE EASY _Milton L. Hanauer_	3.00
_____	CHESS PROBLEMS FOR BEGINNERS _edited by Fred Reinfeld_	2.00
_____	CHESS SECRETS REVEALED _Fred Reinfeld_	2.00
_____	CHESS TACTICS FOR BEGINNERS _edited by Fred Reinfeld_	4.00
_____	CHESS THEORY & PRACTICE _Morry & Mitchell_	2.00
_____	HOW TO WIN AT CHECKERS _Fred Reinfeld_	3.00
_____	1001 BRILLIANT WAYS TO CHECKMATE _Fred Reinfeld_	4.00
_____	1001 WINNING CHESS SACRIFICES & COMBINATIONS _Fred Reinfeld_	4.00
_____	SOVIET CHESS _Edited by R. G. Wade_	3.00

COOKERY & HERBS

____ CULPEPER'S HERBAL REMEDIES *Dr. Nicholas Culpeper*	3.00
____ FAST GOURMET COOKBOOK *Poppy Cannon*	2.50
____ GINSENG The Myth & The Truth *Joseph P. Hou*	3.00
____ HEALING POWER OF HERBS *May Bethel*	4.00
____ HEALING POWER OF NATURAL FOODS *May Bethel*	5.00
____ HERB HANDBOOK *Dawn MacLeod*	3.00
____ HERBS FOR HEALTH—How to Grow & Use Them *Louise Evans Doole*	4.00
____ HOME GARDEN COOKBOOK—Delicious Natural Food Recipes *Ken Kraft*	3.00
____ MEDICAL HERBALIST *edited by Dr. J. R. Yemm*	3.00
____ VEGETABLE GARDENING FOR BEGINNERS *Hugh Wiberg*	2.00
____ VEGETABLES FOR TODAY'S GARDENS *R. Milton Carleton*	2.00
____ VEGETARIAN COOKERY *Janet Walker*	4.00
____ VEGETARIAN COOKING MADE EASY & DELECTABLE *Veronica Vezza*	3.00
____ VEGETARIAN DELIGHTS—A Happy Cookbook for Health *K. R. Mehta*	2.00
____ VEGETARIAN GOURMET COOKBOOK *Joyce McKinnel*	3.00

GAMBLING & POKER

____ ADVANCED POKER STRATEGY & WINNING PLAY *A. D. Livingston*	5.00
____ HOW TO WIN AT DICE GAMES *Skip Frey*	3.00
____ HOW TO WIN AT POKER *Terence Reese & Anthony T. Watkins*	5.00
____ WINNING AT CRAPS *Dr. Lloyd T. Commins*	4.00
____ WINNING AT GIN *Chester Wander & Cy Rice*	3.00
____ WINNING AT POKER—An Expert's Guide *John Archer*	5.00
____ WINNING AT 21—An Expert's Guide *John Archer*	5.00
____ WINNING POKER SYSTEMS *Norman Zadeh*	3.00

HEALTH

____ BEE POLLEN *Lynda Lyngheim & Jack Scagnetti*	3.00
____ DR. LINDNER'S SPECIAL WEIGHT CONTROL METHOD *P. G. Lindner, M.D.*	2.00
____ HELP YOURSELF TO BETTER SIGHT *Margaret Darst Corbett*	3.00
____ HOW TO IMPROVE YOUR VISION *Dr. Robert A. Kraskin*	3.00
____ HOW YOU CAN STOP SMOKING PERMANENTLY *Ernest Caldwell*	3.00
____ MIND OVER PLATTER *Peter G. Lindner, M.D.*	3.00
____ NATURE'S WAY TO NUTRITION & VIBRANT HEALTH *Robert J. Scrutton*	3.00
____ NEW CARBOHYDRATE DIET COUNTER *Patti Lopez-Pereira*	2.00
____ QUICK & EASY EXERCISES FOR FACIAL BEAUTY *Judy Smith-deal*	2.00
____ QUICK & EASY EXERCISES FOR FIGURE BEAUTY *Judy Smith-deal*	2.00
____ REFLEXOLOGY *Dr. Maybelle Segal*	4.00
____ REFLEXOLOGY FOR GOOD HEALTH *Anna Kaye & Don C. Matchan*	5.00
____ 30 DAYS TO BEAUTIFUL LEGS *Dr. Marc Selner*	3.00
____ YOU CAN LEARN TO RELAX *Dr. Samuel Gutwirth*	3.00
____ YOUR ALLERGY—What To Do About It *Allan Knight, M.D.*	3.00

HOBBIES

____ BEACHCOMBING FOR BEGINNERS *Norman Hickin*	2.00
____ BLACKSTONE'S MODERN CARD TRICKS *Harry Blackstone*	3.00
____ BLACKSTONE'S SECRETS OF MAGIC *Harry Blackstone*	3.00
____ COIN COLLECTING FOR BEGINNERS *Burton Hobson & Fred Reinfeld*	3.00
____ ENTERTAINING WITH ESP *Tony 'Doc' Shiels*	2.00
____ 400 FASCINATING MAGIC TRICKS YOU CAN DO *Howard Thurston*	4.00
____ HOW I TURN JUNK INTO FUN AND PROFIT *Sari*	3.00
____ HOW TO WRITE A HIT SONG & SELL IT *Tommy Boyce*	7.00
____ JUGGLING MADE EASY *Rudolf Dittrich*	3.00
____ MAGIC FOR ALL AGES *Walter Gibson*	4.00
____ MAGIC MADE EASY *Byron Wels*	2.00
____ STAMP COLLECTING FOR BEGINNERS *Burton Hobson*	3.00

HORSE PLAYERS' WINNING GUIDES

____ BETTING HORSES TO WIN *Les Conklin*	3.00
____ ELIMINATE THE LOSERS *Bob McKnight*	3.00
____ HOW TO PICK WINNING HORSES *Bob McKnight*	5.00
____ HOW TO WIN AT THE RACES *Sam (The Genius) Lewin*	5.00
____ HOW YOU CAN BEAT THE RACES *Jack Kavanagh*	5.00
____ MAKING MONEY AT THE RACES *David Barr*	5.00

_____ PAYDAY AT THE RACES *Les Conklin*	3.00
_____ SMART HANDICAPPING MADE EASY *William Bauman*	·5.00
_____ SUCCESS AT THE HARNESS RACES *Barry Meadow*	5.00
_____ WINNING AT THE HARNESS RACES—An Expert's Guide *Nick Cammarano*	5.00

HUMOR

_____ HOW TO BE A COMEDIAN FOR FUN & PROFIT *King & Laufer*	2.00
_____ HOW TO FLATTEN YOUR TUSH *Coach Marge Reardon*	2.00
_____ HOW TO MAKE LOVE TO YOURSELF *Ron Stevens & Joy Grdnic*	3.00
_____ JOKE TELLER'S HANDBOOK *Bob Orben*	4.00
_____ JOKES FOR ALL OCCASIONS *Al Schock*	4.00
_____ 2000 NEW LAUGHS FOR SPEAKERS *Bob Orben*	5.00
_____ 2,500 JOKES TO START 'EM LAUGHING *Bob Orben*	5.00

HYPNOTISM

_____ ADVANCED TECHNIQUES OF HYPNOSIS *Melvin Powers*	3.00
_____ BRAINWASHING AND THE CULTS *Paul A. Verdier, Ph.D.*	3.00
_____ CHILDBIRTH WITH HYPNOSIS *William S. Kroger, M.D.*	5.00
_____ HOW TO SOLVE Your Sex Problems with Self-Hypnosis *Frank S. Caprio, M.D.*	5.00
_____ HOW TO STOP SMOKING THRU SELF-HYPNOSIS *Leslie M. LeCron*	3.00
_____ HOW TO USE AUTO-SUGGESTION EFFECTIVELY *John Duckworth*	3.00
_____ HOW YOU CAN BOWL BETTER USING SELF-HYPNOSIS *Jack Heise*	4.00
_____ HOW YOU CAN PLAY BETTER GOLF USING SELF-HYPNOSIS *Jack Heise*	3.00
_____ HYPNOSIS AND SELF-HYPNOSIS *Bernard Hollander, M.D.*	5.00
_____ HYPNOTISM *(Originally published in 1893) Carl Sextus*	5.00
_____ HYPNOTISM & PSYCHIC PHENOMENA *Simeon Edmunds*	4.00
_____ HYPNOTISM MADE EASY *Dr. Ralph Winn*	3.00
_____ HYPNOTISM MADE PRACTICAL *Louis Orton*	5.00
_____ HYPNOTISM REVEALED *Melvin Powers*	2.00
_____ HYPNOTISM TODAY *Leslie LeCron and Jean Bordeaux, Ph.D.*	5.00
_____ MODERN HYPNOSIS *Lesley Kuhn & Salvatore Russo, Ph.D.*	5.00
_____ NEW CONCEPTS OF HYPNOSIS *Bernard C. Gindes, M.D.*	**7.00**
_____ NEW SELF-HYPNOSIS *Paul Adams*	5.00
_____ POST-HYPNOTIC INSTRUCTIONS—Suggestions for Therapy *Arnold Furst*	5.00
_____ PRACTICAL GUIDE TO SELF-HYPNOSIS *Melvin Powers*	3.00
_____ PRACTICAL HYPNOTISM *Philip Magonet, M.D.*	3.00
_____ SECRETS OF HYPNOTISM *S. J. Van Pelt, M.D.*	5.00
_____ SELF-HYPNOSIS A Conditioned-Response Technique *Laurence Sparks*	7.00
_____ SELF-HYPNOSIS Its Theory, Technique & Application *Melvin Powers*	3.00
_____ THERAPY THROUGH HYPNOSIS *edited by Raphael H. Rhodes*	5.00

JUDAICA

_____ MODERN ISRAEL *Lily Edelman*	2.00
_____ SERVICE OF THE HEART *Evelyn Garfiel, Ph.D.*	7.00
_____ STORY OF ISRAEL IN COINS *Jean & Maurice Gould*	2.00
_____ STORY OF ISRAEL IN STAMPS *Maxim & Gabriel Shamir*	1.00
_____ TONGUE OF THE PROPHETS *Robert St. John*	5.00

JUST FOR WOMEN

_____ COSMOPOLITAN'S GUIDE TO MARVELOUS MEN Fwd. by *Helen Gurley Brown*	3.00
_____ COSMOPOLITAN'S HANG-UP HANDBOOK Foreword by *Helen Gurley Brown*	4.00
_____ COSMOPOLITAN'S LOVE BOOK—A Guide to Ecstasy in Bed	5.00
_____ COSMOPOLITAN'S NEW ETIQUETTE GUIDE Fwd. by *Helen Gurley Brown*	4.00
_____ I AM A COMPLEAT WOMAN *Doris Hagopian & Karen O'Connor Sweeney*	3.00
_____ JUST FOR WOMEN—A Guide to the Female Body *Richard E. Sand, M.D.*	5.00
_____ NEW APPROACHES TO SEX IN MARRIAGE *John E. Eichenlaub, M.D.*	3.00
_____ SEXUALLY ADEQUATE FEMALE *Frank S. Caprio, M.D.*	3.00
_____ SEXUALLY FULFILLED WOMAN *Dr. Rachel Copelan*	5.00
_____ YOUR FIRST YEAR OF MARRIAGE *Dr. Tom McGinnis*	3.00

MARRIAGE, SEX & PARENTHOOD

_____ ABILITY TO LOVE *Dr. Allan Fromme*	6.00
_____ GUIDE TO SUCCESSFUL MARRIAGE *Drs. Albert Ellis & Robert Harper*	5.00
_____ HOW TO RAISE AN EMOTIONALLY HEALTHY, HAPPY CHILD *A. Ellis*	5.00
_____ SEX WITHOUT GUILT *Albert Ellis, Ph.D.*	5.00
_____ SEXUALLY ADEQUATE MALE *Frank S. Caprio, M.D.*	3.00

_____ SEXUALLY FULFILLED MAN *Dr. Rachel Copelan*	5.00
_____ STAYING IN LOVE *Dr. Norton F. Kristy*	7.00

MELVIN POWERS' MAIL ORDER LIBRARY

_____ HOW TO GET RICH IN MAIL ORDER *Melvin Powers*	15.00
_____ HOW TO WRITE A GOOD ADVERTISEMENT *Victor O. Schwab*	15.00
_____ MAIL ORDER MADE EASY *J. Frank Brumbaugh*	10.00
_____ U.S. MAIL ORDER SHOPPER'S GUIDE *Susan Spitzer*	10.00

METAPHYSICS & OCCULT

_____ BOOK OF TALISMANS, AMULETS & ZODIACAL GEMS *William Pavitt*	5.00
_____ CONCENTRATION—A Guide to Mental Mastery *Mouni Sadhu*	5.00
_____ CRITIQUES OF GOD *Edited by Peter Angeles*	7.00
_____ EXTRA-TERRESTRIAL INTELLIGENCE—The First Encounter	6.00
_____ FORTUNE TELLING WITH CARDS *P. Foli*	4.00
_____ HANDWRITING ANALYSIS MADE EASY *John Marley*	5.00
_____ HANDWRITING TELLS *Nadya Olyanova*	7.00
_____ HOW TO INTERPRET DREAMS, OMENS & FORTUNE TELLING SIGNS *Gettings*	3.00
_____ HOW TO UNDERSTAND YOUR DREAMS *Geoffrey A. Dudley*	3.00
_____ ILLUSTRATED YOGA *William Zorn*	3.00
_____ IN DAYS OF GREAT PEACE *Mouni Sadhu*	3.00
_____ LSD—THE AGE OF MIND *Bernard Roseman*	2.00
_____ MAGICIAN—His Training and Work *W. E. Butler*	3.00
_____ MEDITATION *Mouni Sadhu*	7.00
_____ MODERN NUMEROLOGY *Morris C. Goodman*	5.00
_____ NUMEROLOGY—ITS FACTS AND SECRETS *Ariel Yvon Taylor*	3.00
_____ NUMEROLOGY MADE EASY *W. Mykian*	5.00
_____ PALMISTRY MADE EASY *Fred Gettings*	5.00
_____ PALMISTRY MADE PRACTICAL *Elizabeth Daniels Squire*	5.00
_____ PALMISTRY SECRETS REVEALED *Henry Frith*	4.00
_____ PROPHECY IN OUR TIME *Martin Ebon*	2.50
_____ PSYCHOLOGY OF HANDWRITING *Nadya Olyanova*	5.00
_____ SUPERSTITION—Are You Superstitious? *Eric Maple*	2.00
_____ TAROT *Mouni Sadhu*	8.00
_____ TAROT OF THE BOHEMIANS *Papus*	5.00
_____ WAYS TO SELF-REALIZATION *Mouni Sadhu*	3.00
_____ WHAT YOUR HANDWRITING REVEALS *Albert E. Hughes*	3.00
_____ WITCHCRAFT, MAGIC & OCCULTISM—A Fascinating History *W. B. Crow*	5.00
_____ WITCHCRAFT—THE SIXTH SENSE *Justine Glass*	5.00
_____ WORLD OF PSYCHIC RESEARCH *Hereward Carrington*	2.00

SELF-HELP & INSPIRATIONAL

_____ DAILY POWER FOR JOYFUL LIVING *Dr. Donald Curtis*	5.00
_____ DYNAMIC THINKING *Melvin Powers*	2.00
_____ GREATEST POWER IN THE UNIVERSE *U. S. Andersen*	5.00
_____ GROW RICH WHILE YOU SLEEP *Ben Sweetland*	3.00
_____ GROWTH THROUGH REASON *Albert Ellis, Ph.D.*	4.00
_____ GUIDE TO PERSONAL HAPPINESS *Albert Ellis, Ph.D. & Irving Becker, Ed. D.*	5.00
_____ HELPING YOURSELF WITH APPLIED PSYCHOLOGY *R. Henderson*	2.00
_____ HOW TO ATTRACT GOOD LUCK *A. H. Z. Carr*	5.00
_____ HOW TO BE GREAT *Dr. Donald Curtis*	5.00
_____ HOW TO DEVELOP A WINNING PERSONALITY *Martin Panzer*	5.00
_____ HOW TO DEVELOP AN EXCEPTIONAL MEMORY *Young & Gibson*	5.00
_____ HOW TO LIVE WITH A NEUROTIC *Albert Ellis, Ph. D.*	5.00
_____ HOW TO OVERCOME YOUR FEARS *M. P. Leahy, M.D.*	3.00
_____ HOW TO SUCCEED *Brian Adams*	7.00
_____ HOW YOU CAN HAVE CONFIDENCE AND POWER *Les Giblin*	5.00
_____ HUMAN PROBLEMS & HOW TO SOLVE THEM *Dr. Donald Curtis*	5.00
_____ I CAN *Ben Sweetland*	7.00
_____ I WILL *Ben Sweetland*	3.00
_____ LEFT-HANDED PEOPLE *Michael Barsley*	5.00
_____ MAGIC IN YOUR MIND *U. S. Andersen*	6.00
_____ MAGIC OF THINKING BIG *Dr. David J. Schwartz*	3.00
_____ MAGIC POWER OF YOUR MIND *Walter M. Germain*	5.00

*The books listed above can be obtained from your book dealer or directly from
Melvin Powers. When ordering, please remit $1.00 postage for the first book
and 50¢ for each additional book.*

Melvin Powers

12015 Sherman Road, No. Hollywood, California 91605